er

Research and Perspectives in Long

Spring

Berlin
Heidelberg
New York
Barcelona
Hong Kong
London
Milan
Paris
Singapore
Tokyo

J.-M. Robine B. Forette
C. Franceschi M. Allard (Eds.)

The Paradoxes
of Longevity

With 34 Figures and 10 Tables

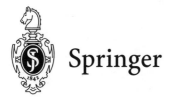

Springer

JEAN-MARIE ROBINE
Equipe INSERM Démographie et Santé
Val d'Aurelle
Parc Euromédecine
F-34298 Montpellier Cedex 5
France

BERNARD FORETTE
Hôpital Sainte Perine
11, rue Chardon-Lagache
F-75016 Paris
France

CLAUDIO FRANCESCHI
INRCA
Via Barelli, 8
I-60100 Ancona
Italy

MICHEL ALLARD
Fondation IPSEN
24, rue Erlanger
F-75781 Paris Cedex 16
France

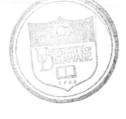

ISBN 3-540-65544-1 Springer-Verlag Berlin Heidelberg New York

Library of Congress Cataloging-in-Publication Data
The paradoxes of longevity / J.-M. Robine ... [et al.] (eds.). p.   cm. – (Research and perspectives in longevity) Includes bibliographical references and index. ISBN 3-540-65544-1 (hc.)   1. Longevity.   I. Robine, Jean-Marie. II. Series.   QP85.P34   1999   612.6'8–dc21

Production: PRO EDIT GmbH, D-69126 Heidelberg
Cover design: design & production, D-69121 Heidelberg
Typesetting: Mitterweger Werksatz GmbH, D-68723 Plankstadt, Germany
SPIN: 10710673   27/3136/SPS – 5 4 3 2 1 0 – Printed in acid-free paper

Preface

An important part of our research work deals with the assessment of change over time. Whatever the measures used, active life expectancy for instance, time series are needed involving at least two points in time. Thus, with this second symposium "The paradoxes of longevity", held in March 1998 and following the first one "Longevity, to the limits and beyond" held in March 1996, we are completing a new series of Fondation IPSEN's "Colloques Médecine et Recherche", a new series which we would want to believe is far from being closed.

When we started our discussion in 1994, the possibility for the Fondation IPSEN of setting up a new prize – the Longevity Prize – and a new series of colloquia dealing with longevity research, research on longevity was not very fashionable! The Fondation IPSEN, convinced that research on longevity was to have a crucial importance for the future, pioneered a representative survey of centenarians in 1990 "In search of the secret of centenarians", and in the early 90s strongly supported the CHRONOS study, the objectives of which were to discover genes associated with extreme longevity. Four years later, in 1998, "research on longevity" seemed fashionable. As attested by the titles of papers in "Science", "Nature" or other journals, the world "longevity" is used constantly more often worldwide. But, it is not only fashionable if we refer to the large number of possible candidates for the last selection of the Longevity Prize.

The Longevity Prize is already a time series: In 1996, Caleb Finch got it for his work on the genetics of longevity, in 1997, Vaino Kannisto for his work on the demography of the oldest old and in 1998, Roy Walford for his work on the effect of calorie restriction on longevity. We wish the winners of the prize a long life and a slow senescence process without dependence on a care provider, what Aristote called Eugeria and what we call today a healthy active aging.

Living longer? What is the price of a longer life? senescence, calorie restriction, "waiting mode", French cuisine ... increasing the length of life without increasing the quality of the years lived is a hollow prize. According to the WHO, the goal to be reached for the 21st century is no longer increasing life expectancy or reducing mortality levels, but increasing health expectancy and fighting disabilities and senescence. On this topic and through the examination of various paradoxes, whether we are "complicationists" or "simplificationists", we have learned a lot during this symposium: how some species achieve great longevity with minimal senescence, or again new research avenues to explain the onset of the major age-related pathologies such as dementia, osteoporosis, and athero-sclerosis.

JEAN-MARIE ROBINE
BERNARD FORETTE
CLAUDIO FRANCESCHI
MICHEL ALLARD

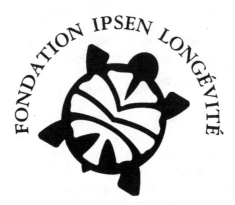

Acknowledgements: The editors wish to thank Mary Lynn Gage and Isabelle Romieu for editorial assistance and Jacqueline Mervaillie for the organization of the meeting in Paris.

Contents

Contributors

CAREY, JAMES R.
Department of Entomology, University of California, Davis, CA 95616-8584, USA

CARRIÈRE, Y.
Simon Fraser University, Vancouver, Canada

FINCH, CALEB E.
Division of Neurogerontology, Ethel Percy Andrus Gerontology Center, University Park, MC-0191 3715 McClintok, Los Angeles, CA 90089-0191, USA

FORETTE, BERNARD
Hôpital Sainte Perine, 11, rue Chardon-Lagache, 75781 Paris, France

FRIEDMAN, HOWARD
Department of Psychology, University of California, Riverside, CA 92521-1426, USA

GERBER, MARIETTE
Groupe d'Épidémiologie Métabolique, Centre de Recherches en Cancérologie, INSERM-CRLC, 34298 Montpellier Cedex 5, France

GREINER, L. H.
Sanders-Brown Center on Aging, College of Medicine, University of Kentucky, 101 Sanders Brown Bldg, Lexington, KY 40536-0230, USA

HORIUCHI, SHIRO
Laboratory of Populations, Rockefeller University, 1230 York Avenue, Box 20, New York, NY 10021-6399, USA

HWANG, E. H.
Department of Physiology, The University of Texas Health Sciences Center, 7703 Floyd Curl Drive, San Antonio, TX 78284-7756, USA

Kemper, S. J.
Psychology Department, University of Kansas, Lawrence, KS, USA

Lee, D. Y.
Department of Physiology, The University of Texas Health Sciences Center,
7703 Floyd Curl Drive, San Antonio, TX 78284-7756, USA

Légaré, Jacques
Department of Demography, University of Montreal, PO Box 6128 Succ.
Centre ville, Montreal, Quebec H3C 3J7, Canada

Lim, B. O.
Department of Physiology, The University of Texas Health Sciences Center,
7703 Floyd Curl Drive, San Antonio, TX 78284-7756, USA

Martin, George M.
Department of Pathology, University of Washington, Health Sciences Building
K-543, 1959 NE Pacific Avenue, PO Box 357470, Seattle, WA,
98195-7470, USA

Mortimer, J. A.
Institute on Aging, University of South Florida, Tampa, FL, USA

Nanajakkara, N.
Sanders-Brown Center on Aging, College of Medicine,
University of Kentucky, 101 Sanders Brown Bldg, Lexington, KY 40536-0230,
USA

Smith, David W. E.
Department of Pathology, Buehler Center on Aging, Northwestern University
Medical School, 750 North Lake Shore Drive, #601, Chicago, IL 60611-3008,
USA

Snowdon, David A.
The Sanders-Brown Center on Aging, University of Kentucky, 101 Sanders
Brown Bldg, Lexington, KY 40536-0230, USA

Wilmoth, John R.
Department of Demography, University of California, 2232 Piedmont Avenue,
Berkeley, CA 94720-2120, USA

Yu, Byung Pal
Department of Physiology, The University of Texas Health Sciences Center,
7703 Floyd Curl Drive, San Antonio, TX 78284-7756, USA

Longevity Without Aging: Possible Examples

C. E. Finch[1]

The progressive increases in human life spans to unprecedented advanced ages throughout the world diverge from the historical premise that each species has a fixed maximum life span, due to a hard-wired genetic program. The record human life span of 122 years (Jeanne Calment) falls in the middle range of life spans of other multicellular species. As the most longevous among mammals, our life spans dwarf those of laboratory rodents by 30-fold (Finch 1990). Most other phyla also include species that differ widely, by powers of 10, in life spans (Fig. 1). The total range of life spans for individual organisms is nearly a million-fold, from yeast to conifers. One measure of the rate of senescence in a population is the time required for mortality rate doubling (MRD; Finch et al. 1990), which ranges at least 1,000-fold (Table 1). This diversity of life spans and rates of senescence within phyla suggests that the type of body plan (bauplan) itself does not set stringent limits on the range of life spans that may be evolved.

The individual ages of very long-lived plants and animals can sometimes be determined by annual growth rings, which have been used to establish convincingly that trees of many genera grow productively for a millennium or more, thereby exceeding any record in multicellular animals by 5- to 20-fold. The record individual life span for any tree is that of a Great Basin bristlecone pine (*Pinus longaeva*) of 4,862 years in the high Nevada mountains (Lanner 1998)[2]. Much is known about the natural history of the Great Basin bristlecone pine, from studies by Ronald M. Lanner and his then graduate student, Kristina F. Connor. This carefully obtained and conservatively interpreted body of work is not widely known to biomedical gerontologists.

The key finding of Lanner and Connor is that reproduction does not decline with aging in trees up to at least 4,713 years. These conclusions are based on observations made under controlled laboratory conditions of seed weight (Fig. 2A),

---

[1] Neurogerontology Division, Andrus Gerontology Center and Department of Biological Sciences, University of Southern California, Los Angeles, CA 90089-0191, USA

[2] The Great Basin was in part formed during the last glacial age (Wisconsonian), about 20,000 years ago, in the present state of Nevada and its neighbors, and is presently a semidesert plane bounded by high mountains on the west and east, and broken by numerous other smaller ranges. These complex montaine ecosystems support about 22 species of conifer. The designation of *Pinus longaeva* as the Great Basin bristlecone pine is made to distinguish it from its close relative, the Rocky Mountain bristlecone, *Pinus aristata*, which probably does not achieve as great ages. Lanner (1984) cautions that this distinction was not made in the early literature (before 1980).

J.-M. Robine et al. (Eds.)
Research and Perspectives in Longevity
The Paradoxes of Longevity
© Springer-Verlag Berlin Heidelberg New York 1999

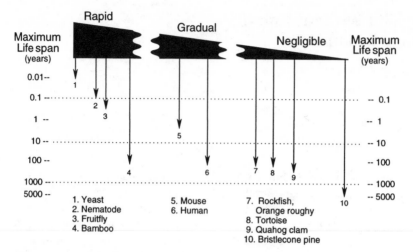

1. Yeast
2. Nematode
3. Fruitfly
4. Bamboo

5. Mouse
6. Human

7. Rockfish,
   Orange roughy
8. Tortoise
9. Quahog clam
10. Bristlecone pine

Fig. 1. A sample of species that differ widely in longevity (total life span from zygote to oldest adult in years) and the rate of senescence in adults (semi-quantitative scale ranging from rapid to gradual to negligible senescence). Maximum life spans depends on husbandry conditions (temperature, nutrition). Sources of data are found in Finch (1990), except as indicated.

Rapid senescence. Yeast (*Saccharomyces cerevisae*), 2–4 days during asexual budding. Nematode (*Caenorhabditis elegans*), 30 days. Fruitfly (*Drosophila melanogaster*), 60 days. Pacific salmon, 3–6 years (*Onchorynchus*). Vascular plants: thick-stemmed bamboo (*Phyllostachys bambusoides, P. henonis*) 120 years. *Puya raimondii* (related to the pineapple), 150 years.

Gradual senescence. Mouse (*Mus musculus*), 4,2 years (1541 days). Human (Jeanne Calment), 122.4 years (Robine and Allard 1998).

Negligible senescence. Fish: rockfish (*Sebastes aleutianus*), 140 years; orange roughy (*Hoplostethus atlanticus*), 140 years (Fenton et al. 1991; Smith et al. 1991); warty oreo (*Allocyttus verrucosus*), >130 years (Stewart et al. 1992); sturgeon (*Acipenser fulvescens*), 152 years; Tortoise (*Geochelone gigantea*), 150 years; Bivalve mollusc: ocean quahog (*Artica islandica* 220 years. Great Basin bristlecone pine (*Pinus longaeva*), 4,862 years – however, because ring-dating often underestimates, it is likely that the true ages are >5,000 years (Lanner, 1998). Inclusion of clonal, asexual reproducing species, e.g. clones of the creosote bush (*Larrea tridentata*) and other asexually reproducing plants and animal species, would extend the upper range of postzygotic individual life spans to >10,000 years

seed germination (Fig. 2B), and seedling growth rates (Fig. 2C), which are from the Methuselah Grove (Conner and Lanner 1989, 1991). Nor did age alter the annual vegetative growth of shoots (Fig. 3A, B), or the growth of cambium, or shoot microstructure (Conner and Lanner 1989).

Moreover, parental tree age did not alter the frequency of abnormal germinants (putative mutations), as detected by atypical colors and shapes of the germinants, all of which failed to grow further. As shown in Figure 2D, the highest incidence of abnormalities was 1% from a sample of the oldest trees in the Methuselah Grove (n = 5 trees, aged 1,995–4,713 years, average 3,062 years). Note that a similar sample from the Mammoth grove (n = 5, aged 1,014–1,623 years, average age 1,239 years) had no mutations. It is possible that some individual trees have preferentially accumulated mutations, because two of the abnormal germinants from the Mammoth Grove came from the same tree, aged 823 years.

Table 1. Life spans and Mortality Rate Doubling (MRD) Times[a]

Species	Life span (years)	MRD (years)
Yeast (budding)	0.01	0.004
Fruitfly	0.3	0.03
Honeybee		
Worker, summer	0.2	0.02
winter	0.9	0.03, after leaving hive
Queen	>5	>1
Nematode	0.15	0.03
Mouse	3	0.25
Herring gull	49	3
Human	15–80	8
	>100	>16
Lake sturgeon	150	10
Bristlecone pine	4,862	?

[a] Most of these data were quoted from Finch (1990) and Finch et al. (1990). The MRD of human centenarians must be at least twice as long as that observed before the mean life span, because mortality rates approach a maximum of 0.5/year after 105 years (Vaupel 1997 a). There are too few survivors at highly advanced ages in human, fish, and conifer population to calculate meaningful statistic on the MRD.

In interpreting these data, it is important to recall that germinal tissues of trees, like other plants, differentiate just before seasonal reproduction, from undifferentiated (totipotent) meristematic cells. This pattern of reproductive development differs from that found in most (but not all) animals, in which the germ cells are set aside early in development. It would be of high interest to know seed viability in other trees of many genera that grow productively for a millennium or more. The continuing reproduction of these remarkable trees is a powerful counter example to the many other sexually reproducing species of perennial plants and animals that show reproductive declines (Finch 1990). Molecular and cellular studies of gametogenesis and development are feasible, given the ample availability of materials that can be sampled without harming these trees.

Death of these ancient trees seems to be due to external hazards including fire, soil erosion, and boring insects that enable fungal rot, as described in enjoyable passages quoted from Lanner (1984) – *"Trees of the Great Basin"* (pp. 27–28).

"Why does Great Basin bristlecone pine live so long? Perhaps the proper question is, why does it take so long to die? Research has not yet seriously sought the answer, but clues abound. Edmund Schulman was the first to point out that very old trees in the arid West live in extremely harsh environments, and he proposed that adversity begets longevity. He and others suggested several reasons for this: plants are more widely scattered in adverse sites, resulting in lessened competition; less vegetation means few fires entering the stand from outside; slower growth on these sites results in denser, more resinous, more decay-resistant wood; and dry air and soil retard the growth of decay organisms. All of these factors probably have some influence in prolonging the life of an old tree.

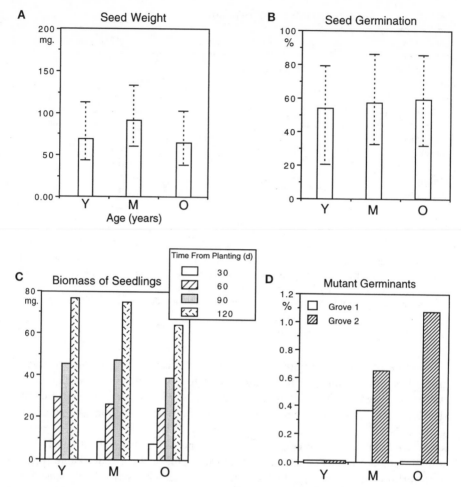

Fig. 2 A–D. Seed and seedling characteristics of aging Great Basin bristlecone pine. Data are graphed from tables of Connor and Lanner (1991) for Methuselah Grove, which had the oldest specimens. Three age groups (n = 5 each) are Y, young (average 3,062 years, range 700–1,269 years); M, middle aged (1,732 years; range 1,558–1,945 years); O, oldest (3,062 years; range 1,995–4,713 years). The bars show the means and the range of values in panels **A** and **B**. Panel **C** shows the growth of seedlings (oven-dried biomass) of two individuals from each age group from the Methuselah and Mammoth Groves (youngest; median ages; oldest). Panel **D** shows the frequency of abnormal germinants from both groves

The oldest bristlecone yet examined was felled in Wheeler Peak [near Las Vegas, Nevada] in 1964: it had 4,844 rings[2] in a section cut from its base, and its total age was estimated at 4,900 years. It was cut down while still alive, so we will never know how long it might have lived. Yet, left alone this tree too would eventually have died. How? It is not known whether every ancient trees finally "wear out",

---

[2] This record is superseded by ring counts from tree WPN-114 at 4,862 years, again likely to be an underestimate (Lanner 1997, 1998).

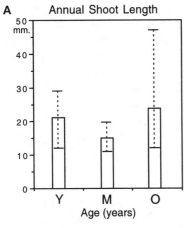
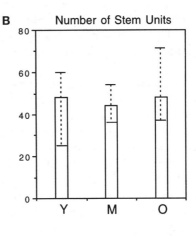

Fig. 3 A, B. Shoot growth characteristics of aging Great Basin bristlecone pine. Data of the annually growing new shoots are graphed from Table 3 (Methuselah Grove) Connor and Lanner (1989). Ages differ slightly from data shown in Fig. 2: five youngest (883–1219 years); five median aged (1564–1944 years); five oldest (2,863–4256 years). The bars show the means and the range of values

or if death requires a discrete and decisive event for its consummation. But even if a tree could avoid fire, lightning and disease, it would some day lose its anchorage through the exposure of its roots by soil erosion. Indeed, the exposed roots of trees of known age have been used to estimate rates of mass-wasting, the geological process that wears away mountains.

But the tree continues to live. Eventually some of its roots perish, perhaps through the slow but steady work of parasitic fungi, or because the erosion of soil gradually uncovers its roots, causing them to dry out and die. Consequently, those sectors of the trunk and the branches above them, that are connected by the alignment of their fibers to the dead roots, also die. Soil water continues to flow into the sapwood leading from healthy roots, up the trunk, to needled limbs; and the photosynthate manufactured in those needles moves downwards, within the phloem, or inner bark, of the limbs into the healthy roots.

As dead strips of trunk dry out, their bark sloughs off, revealing bare wood. Over the centuries root death continue, until a great trunk may consist of a cylindrical expanse of weathered wood traversed by one or more sinuous strips of living bark connecting the occasional live limb to the occasional live root. Beneath that bark the cambium keeps producing a new layer of wood each year, though it be a mere few cells thick. Such a tree is well along the downward slide.

Some claim that the "lifeline" of a functioning trunk results from an evolved response, on the part of the tree, aimed at adjusting the amount of cambial tissue it can afford to sustain. But this makes virtue of necessity – to die slowly is not an adaptation to one's environment. In the slow-motion existence of a millenarian bristlecone pine the shrinking circumference of living cambium merely marks the slow progress of death from the roots up."

But how do the bristlecone seeds get up to the high altitude locations where they can achieve great ages? In fact, wind-dispersed seed, more typical of pines at lower altitudes, rarely reaches higher altitudes. It turns out that the seeding of bristlecone pine stands at higher elevations depends on Clark's nutcracker, a bird that stores (caches) seeds in these stark locations (Lanner 1988, 1996). Further, I suggest that the extreme life spans at higher altitudes are an adventitious outcome of the evolution of seed-caching behavior, which thereby accessed a new niche for the bristlecone pine and increased its potential life span. One may consider that the recent expansion of human life spans (Vaupel 1997 a, b) parallels that of bristlecones at high altitude, and may be due, in our case, to improvements of hygiene and nutrition that adventitiously favored greater life spans.

Other candidates for negligible senescence are certain deep-dwelling fish that live for at least 140 years, according to otolith and radioisotopic dating (Fenton et al. 1991; Mulligan and Leaman 1992). Other supracentenarians occupy similar habitats: rockfish in the Northwest Pacific (5 species of genus *Sebastes*) (Mulligan and Leaman 1992) and, in the southern hemisphere, the orange roughy (*Hoplostethus atlanticus*, Smith et al. 1995) and warty oreo (*Allocyttus verrucosus*, Stewart et al. 1992, Fig. 1 legend). Readers may have enjoyed the tasty orange roughy that is being harvested towards extinction (Koslow 1997). Study for these fascinating fish has barely begun. The few old rockfish examined had abundant, newly formed eggs (X. de Bruin et al., manuscript in preparation). At all ages, gross pathology is very rare, and the oldest specimens appeared healthy in so far as can be determined from inspection in the gross on the deck of a fishing boat in the north Pacific (Bruce Legman, personal communication). Histopathological studies are being done on aged specimens by Jerry Hendricks (Oregon State University).

Yet other examples of very slow or possibly negligible senescence may be found in turtles and birds, which, by field studies with marked animals and credible anecdotal evidence, are in the upper range of human life spans (Gibbons 1987). A famous specimen of Marion's tortoise (*Geochelone gigantea*; formerly designated *Testudo sumerii*) was observed for more than a century at a British fort on the island of Mauritius, but its reputed age of >150 years (Flower 1937; Comfort 1979) is not unquestioned. Much more convincing examples are at hand from several ongoing longitudinal (mark-recapture) studies of feral turtles, e.g. those conducted in the E.S. George Reserve of the Savannah River Ecology Laboratory (Aiken, South Carolina) (Congdon and Gibbons 1996) and near Stump Lake, a backwater of the Illinois River (Tucker and Moll 1997). In Blanding's turtle (*Emydoidea blandingi*), a group older than 55 years (n = 9) had a 60 % greater reproductive rate than a group aged 20–30 years (n = 12, Congdon and van Loben Sels 1993). Similarly, the red-eared turtle (*Trachemys scripta elegans*) does not show any indications of declining egg production or other signs of reproductive senescence (Trucker and Moll 1997). These and other studies are collecting a formidable data base that will allow probing analysis of reproductive histories and mortality rates as a function of reproduction at advanced ages.

Some birds also appear to age very slowly, with long MRDs (Finch et al. 1990) and life spans that approach the human (Finch 1990; Holmes and Austad 1995). It is striking that no bird or reptile is known that has as short a life span or as clear a presentation of tissue degeneration as found in senescent laboratory rodents. Moreover, birds have normal blood glucose of 250–350 mg/dl, in the range of uncorrected diabetics, and core temperatures of 39–41 °C (Holmes and Austad 1995; Finch 1990). By thermodynamics, the elevated glucose and temperature should cause extensive nonenzymatic oxidation of proteins. But, there are almost no data on biochemical aging of birds. Because avian fibroblasts are more resistant to oxygen toxicity than those from mammals (Ogburn et al. 1998), birds may have evolved unique antioxidant mechanisms that allow great longevity despite their feverish metabolism.

There are few data on mortality rates at advanced ages in animals and plants, which, for animals, would require large captive populations (which do not exist) or difficult banding and recapture studies from natural populations. Nonetheless, the existence of a few individuals of great ages is consistent with very slow mortality rate accelerations; for example for conifers that live >1000 years, the MRDs could be >100 years long (Table 1).

However, a very long MRD is not a sufficient criterion for negligible senescence. For example, the acceleration of mortality in human populations slows after the average life span, so that by the age of 105, mortality rates may not increase higher than a maximum of about 50 % per year and may even show small net decreases in successive year groups (Vaupel 1997a). But, this does not mean that human supracentenarians are rejuvenated by living so long. In fact, most centenarians are in a very fragile state. Thus, long MRDs may indicate a negligible state of senescence, but only when there has not been a preceding phase of accelerating mortality in adults and no decline of reproduction or other vital functions. These criteria may be met in certain conifers and fish. Demographic data are still needed to evaluate if mortality rates accelerate at later ages in these species, which is a criterion for senescence at the population level.

Thus we now have a basis for study of how some species achieve great longevity with minimal senescence. While the evolutionary hypothesis of senescence (Rose 1996; Williams 1965; Charlesworth 1995) predicts that the optimization of the reproductive schedule will select against genes with early adverse effects, the hypothesis does not inform about rates of senescence. Nonetheless, population biologists generally conclude from mathematical models that "... senescence always creeps in", in Hamilton's trenchant phrase (Hamilton 1966). This reasoning does not predict the apparent negligible senescence of long-lived conifers and fish that maintain reproduction at their most advanced ages. Moreover, it is puzzling that inbred invertebrates, like many other species, include relatively robust individuals that comprise subpopulations with reduced mortality rates at advanced ages (Vaupel 1997a). This diversity is consistent with genetic studies of humans, mice, flies, and worms, which concluded that the heritability of life span is minor, <35 % of its variance (Finch and Tanzi 1997). Although this implies a relatively greater importance of the environment than genes to outcomes of aging, we do not know the role of nonprogrammed developmental variations in cell numbers, for example, that may endow an individual with organ reserves that favor greater longevity.

In summary, the comparative biology of life histories shows the enormous plasticity of the schedule of senescence during evolution. The prospects for continued increase in human life expectancy are of course unknown, but examples from the natural world suggest that no firm limit is built into the human genome. The efforts to modify human aging via drugs, diet, and life style interventions are entirely consistent with the observed plasticity in life histories of numerous other species. A tissue bank is urgently needed to provide specimens of long-lived organisms for study of possible anti-aging mechanisms that permit achievement of great ages. It is of great interest to obtain data on biochemical and cellular changes at advanced ages of diverse species, as well as on cell and molecular turnover. Time is running out on many very long-lived species whose habitats are being destroyed or which are being commercially overexploited, and these rare populations should be included in endangered species efforts (Finch and Ricklefs 1991).

References

Charlesworth B (1995) Evolution in Age-structure Populations, 2nd ed, U Chicago Press

Comfort A (1979) The Biology of Senescence. Edimburg, London: Churchill Livingston. 3rd ed

Congdon JD and van Loben Sels RC (1993) Relationships of reproductive traits and body size with attainment of sexual maturity and age in Blanding's turtles (*Emydoidea blandingi*). J Evol Biol 6:547–557

Congdon JD and Gibbons JW (1996) Structure and dynamics of a turtle community over two decades. In: Long-Term Studies of Vertebrate Communities, Academic Press New York

Connor KF, Lanner RM (1989) Age-related changes in shoot growth components of Great Basin bristlecone pine. Can J Forest Res 19:933–935

Connor KF, Lanner RM (1991) Effects of tree age on pollen, seed, and seedline characteristics in Great Basin bristlecone pine. Bot Gaz 152:107–113

Fenton GE, Short SA, Ritz DA (1991) Age determination of orange roughy *Hoplostethus atlanticus* using ^{210}Pb: ^{226}Ra disequilibria. Marine Biol 109:197–202

Finch CE (1990) Longevity, Senescence, and the Genome, U Chicago Press, Chicago

Finch CE, Ricklefs RE (1991) Age structure of populations (letter). Science 254–799

Finch CE, Tanzi RE (1997) Genetics of aging Science 278:407–411

Finch CE, Pike MC, Witten M (1990) Slow mortality rate accelerations during aging approximate those of humans. Science 249:902–905

Flower SS (1937) Further notes on the duration of life in animals. 3. Reptiles, Proc. Zool. Soc. Lond. Ser A 107:1–39

Gibbons JW (1987) Why do turtles live so long? Bioscience 37:262–269

Hamilton WD (1966) The moulding of senescence by natural selection. J Theoret Biol 12:12–45

Holmes DJ, Austad SN (1995) Birds as animal models for the comparative biology of aging: a prospectus. J Gerontol Biol Sci 50:B59–B66

Koslow JA (1997) Seamounts and the ecology of deep-sea fisheries. Am Scientist 85:168–176

Lanner RM (1984) Trees of the Great Basin. A Natural History. U Nevada Press, Reno

Lanner RM (1988) Dependence of Great Basin bristlecone pine on Clark's nutcracker for regeneration at high elevations. Arctic Alpine Res 20:358–362

Lanner RM (1996) Made for Each Other: A Symbiosis of Birds and Pines Oxford U Press

Lanner RM (1997) Whatever happened to the world's oldest tree. Nevada Mag: May–June, 27–30

Lanner RM (1998) Conifers of California. Cachuma Press, Los Olivos CA

Mulligan TJ, Leaman BM (1992) Length-at-age analysis: can you get what you see? Can J Fish Aquat Sci 49:632–643

Ogburn CE, Austad SN, Holmes DJ, Kiklevich JV, Gollahon K, Ratinovich PS, Martin GM (1998) Cultured renal epithelial cells from birds and mice: enhanced resistance of avian cells to oxidative stress and DNA damage. J Gerontol 53: B287–B293

Robine JM, Allard M (1998) The oldest human. Science 279: 1834–1835

Rose MR (1996) Towards an evolutionary demography. In: Rose MR, Lauder GV eds, Adaptation. San Diego: Academic Press, pp. 96–107

Smith DC, Fenton GE, Robertson SG, Short SA (1995) Age determination and growth of orange roughy (*Hoplostethus atlanticus*): a comparison of annulus counts with radiometric ageing. Can J Fish Aqua Sci 52:391–401

Stewart BD, Fenton GE, Smith DC, Short SA (1992) Validation of otolith-increment age estimates for a deepwater fish species, the warty oreo *Allocyttus verrucosus*, by radiometric analysis. Marine Biol 123:29–38

Tucker JK and Moll D (1997) Growth, reproduction, and survivorship in the red-eared turtle, *Trachemys scripta elegans*, in Illinois with conservation implications. Chelonian Conservation and Biology 2:352–357

Vaupel J (1997a) Trajectories of mortality at advanced ages. In: Wachter K, Finch CE, eds, Biodemography of Aging. Washington; National Academy Press, pp. 17–34

Vaupel JW (1997 b) The average French baby may live 95 or 100 years. In: Longevity: to the Limits and Beyond, J-M Robine, JW Vaupel, B Jeune, M Allard (eds.) Springer, pp. 1–10

Williams QC (1957) Pleiotropy, natural selection and the evolution of senescence. Evolution 11:398–411

Genes that Modulate Longevity and Senescence

G. M. MARTIN[1]

Introduction

Modern gerontology is faced with a major paradox. On the one hand, we have the evolutionary biologists who have concluded that the modulation of longevity and senescence is under highly polygenic controls, that multiple mechanisms are likely to be involved, and that much of the pathology that unfolds is stochastic in origin. Let us refer to members of this camp as the "complificationists." On the other hand, some biologists point to three lines of evidence that seem to challenge this view. They believe that aging may be produced by a small number of major mechanisms, perhaps even a single major mechanism, such as oxidative damage to macromolecules. Let us refer to members of this camp as the "simplificationists." They emphasize the exceedingly well documented observations that calorically restricted rodents have substantially greater life spans than their well fed brethren do. They also point to experiments with nematodes (*Caenorhabditis elegans*) and fruit flies (*Drosophila melanogaster*). In both organisms, simple genetic manipulation, including single gene mutations, may lead to substantial increments of life span. For the case of aging in man, they emphasize research on the Werner syndrome, a recessive progeroid syndrome caused by a mutation in a helicase gene. Homozygotes exhibit an acceleration of multiple aspects of the senescent phenotype, including four of the major geriatric disorders associated with human aging (arteriosclerosis, cancer, diabetes mellitus and osteoporosis).

Where is the truth? In this brief review, I shall present the case for both simplificationists and complificationists. I shall make two conclusions. First of all, it will come as no surprise to conclude that we need much more research before we can assess the relative degree of complexity or simplicity of aging in any animal species. Secondly, we shall conclude that the arguments supporting the complificationist view are more compelling. Perhaps, however, the truth will rest somewhere between the two extreme views.

[1] Department of Pathology, University of Washington, Seattle, WA, 98195-7470, USA.

J.-M. Robine et al. (Eds.)
Research and Perspectives in Longevity
The Paradoxes of Longevity
© Springer-Verlag Berlin Heidelberg New York 1999

The Arguments of the Complificationists

The Evolutionary Biologic Theory of Why We Age

Evolutionary biologists make no claims that they understand *how* we age – i.e., their theories do not inform us as to the underlying proximal mechanisms of aging. They are confident, however, that they have a quite satisfactory answer as to *why* we age. By "they", I refer to a distinguished list of British and American population geneticists and evolutionary biologists that includes JBS Haldane, Peter B. Medawar, William Hamilton, George C. Williams, Brian Charlesworth, TBL Kirkwood, Linda Partridge, Steven N. Austad, Steven C. Stearns, and Michael R. Rose. In recent years, Michael Rose has been particularly vigorous in championing this point of view via his papers (e.g., Rose and Graves 1989), his book (Rose 1991) and his oral presentations at meetings of gerontologists. Steven Austad (1997) developed the basic ideas of the evolutionary biological theory of aging with particular clarity for a general readership. In essence, the theory states that we age because of the decline in the force of natural selection with respect to the age at which alleles reach phenotypic expression. For age-structured populations (i.e., what is observed with species that undergo repeated rounds of reproduction), life history traits, including longevity, are molded by the ecology under which the species evolves. For species that have evolved under conditions of high environmental hazards (predation, infectious disease, accidents, drought, malnutrition), there is strong selective pressure favoring alleles at genetic loci that ensure relatively rapid rates of development and short periods of high fecundity. The consequence is a relatively short life span. Any allele that reaches phenotypic expression late in the life span of those rare individuals who manage to achieve unusual long-term survival does not contribute significantly to the subsequent generations. The genotype of the species continues to be determined by the vastly greater number of individuals representing younger, actively reproducing cohorts. Given a relaxation of such strong selective pressure for early and rapid reproduction (as in the case of an ecology with decreased environmental hazards), there is an opportunity to develop different life history strategies, including those that lead to longer life spans. This theory has found support both in field studies and in the laboratory. Steven Austad (1993) documented a decreased actuarial rate of aging in an insular species of Virginia opossums (*Didelphis virginia*) that evolved in a relatively protective environment, as compared to a sibling parental species continuing its evolution in the more hazardous environment of the mainland. Rose and Charlesworth (1981), Luckinbill and Clare (1985) and Zwaan et al. (1997) have reported laboratory selection experiments consistent with the theory. They involved either indirect or direct selection for increased life span of fruit flies.

Two classes of gene action have been invoked to explain the development of senescence in age-structured populations. The first involves constitutive germ line mutations with neutral effects upon reproductive fitness, but with deleterious effects late in the life span, when these effects escape the force of natural

Table 1. Genetic loci implicated in the pathogenesis of adult-onset dementias of *Homo sapiens*. The onsets of those listed typically range from ages 40–90 years. The relevant gene action therefore escapes the force of natural selection

Gene symbol	Map locus	Gene product	Inheritance	Disorder
APP	21q21.3-q22-.05	β-amyloid precursor protein	AD[a]	FAD
PSEN1	14q24.3	presenilin 1	AD	FAD
PSEN2	1q31-q42	presenilin 2	AD	FAD
APOE	19q13.2	apolipoprotein E	Co-dominant	LOAD
NOTCH3	19p13.2-13.1	notch 3	AD	CADASIL
MAPT	17q21	microtubule-associated protein tau	AD	FTD
?	3	?	AD	FTD

[a] AD autosomal dominant; FAD familial Alzheimer disease; LOAD late-onset (> age 65) Alzheimers disease; CADASIL cerebral autosomal dominant arteriopathy with subcortical infarcts and leukoencephalopathy; FTD frontotemporal dementia.

selection (Medawar 1952). These effects can be expected to be idiosyncratic, with the frequencies varying as functions of genetic drift. They therefore may be regarded as producing "private" modulations of the senescent phenotype (Martin et al. 1996). The prototypic example (originally noted by JBS Haldane) would be some alleles of the Huntington disease mutation. A systematic analysis of the then-known genetic loci of man concluded that mutations or polymorphisms at thousands of genetic loci could be involved in modulating the pathobiology of aging (Martin 1978). Many of them are likely to represent private mutations. My unpublished, preliminary studies of a recent computerized database of genetic loci of man, using a much larger subset of phenotypes, suggest that the 1978 report underestimated the total proportion of the human genome that might be involved. While it is clear from such surveys that variants at a very large number of genes have the potential to modulate patterns of senescence, a particularly dramatic single gene mutation, influencing a large number of senescent phenotypes, involves the Werner helicase locus (Yu et al. 1996). We shall return to this story when we consider the arguments of the "simplificationists," as the existence of this syndrome is often cited as a reason that aging, even in man, may not be so complicated.

A concrete example of the increasing evidence for genetic heterogeneity for a single senescent phenotype comes from research on dementias of late life. There are many genes that increase one's chance of developing dementing illnesses late in the life span (Table 1). Recent examples include notch 3 mutations on chromosome 19 (Joutel et al. 1996) and a mutation in the microtubule-associated protein tau that can cause a form of frontotemporal dementia (Poorkaj et al. 1998; Hutton et al. 1998). More than one autosomal dominant locus may result in a form of frontotemporal dementia, however, as there is at least one family with evidence of a linkage to chromosome 3 (Brown et al. 1995). The neuropathology of dementia of the Alzheimer type (DAT), characterized by neuritic plaques, beta amyloid deposits in plaques and cerebral vessels, neurofibrillary tangles, deficiency of synapses, and neuronal loss, including early involvement of layer 2 of the entorhinal cortex (G'omez-Isla et al. 1996), is quite distinct from those entities, however, and is vastly more prevalent. DAT may in fact have the potential to affect as many as 50 % of human subjects in at least some populations (Evans et al. 1989). Given such information, one might guess that there would be both "private" and "public" genetic modulations of such a common phenotype. Such indeed appears to be the case. Rare autosomal dominant mutations in at least three different loci are necessary and sufficient for the emergence of the disorder. All three loci [APP, coding for the beta amyloid precursor protein on chromosome 21 (Goate et al. 1991); PSENI, coding for the presenilin 1 protein on chromosome 14 (Sherrington et al. 1995; and PSEN2, coding for the highly homologous presenilin 2 protein on chromosome 1 (Levy-Lahad et al. 1995)] appear to influence processing of the beta amyloid precursor protein (reviewed by Hutton and Hardy 1997), providing support for the primacy of beta amyloid metabolism in at least these rare familial forms of DAT. It is virtually certain that other rare "private" mutations exist, as probably less than half of all early-onset forms of familial DAT (onsets arbitrarily considered to be before ages 60 or 65, but usually after age 40) can be explained by the three known mutations (Blacker and Tanzi 1998). One such gene might be on chromosome 12 (Pericak-Vance et al. 1997), although there has so far been no confirmations of linkage to the implicated region of that chromosome. What about forms of DAT associated with public polymorphisms? The now classical example is the apolipoprotein E locus (APOE), characterized by three common alleles (ε 2, 3 and 4) in numerous human populations (Gerdes et al. 1992). APOE ε 4 is now well established as an age-of-onset risk factor for the vastly more prevalent late-onset "sporadic" forms of DAT, as the original publication of Corder et al. (1993) has been confirmed in many independent populations. Other genetic associations have been reported, some of which must await confirmation. A particularly important example is the apparent role of a polymorphism in the promoter region of APOE (Bullido et al. 1998). This study demonstrates the importance of evaluating haplotypes, rather than single site polymorphisms. The delineation of haplotypes would include much more information concerning structural alterations of potential importance to gene regulation.

The Arguments of the Simplificationists

Single Gene Mutations in Nematodes

The simple nematode, Caenorhabditis elegans, has emerged as a leading model organism for the study of animal genetics. The pioneer investigator of the genetics of aging in this organism, Thomas E. Johnson, began his research by demonstrating that a variety of genes can modulate the life span of this organism. He did this by creating recombinant inbred lines from two independent strains and demonstrating a very large range of life spans in segregants (Johnson and Wood

Table 2. Mutations or overexpression (*trk-1*) at several genetic loci of *Caenorhabditis elegans* can result in substantial life span extensions

Gene symbol	Homologous gene	Reference
age-1	phosphatidyl-inositol 3OH kinase	Friedman and Johnson 1988; Morris et al. 1996
daf-2	insulin receptor-like	Kenyon et al. 1993; Kimura et al. 1997
spe-26	actin-associated protein	Van Voorhies 1992; Varkey et al. 1995
clk-1	yeast metabolic regulator *Cat5p*	Ewbank et al. 1997
trk-1	tyrosine kinase receptor	Murakami and Johnson, personal communication

1982). With the exception of the laboratory of Robert Shmookler-Reis (Ebert et al. 1996), there has been no systematic follow-up of that interesting study. Instead, the attention of essentially all investigators interested in the genetics of longevity in these worms has been directed to single gene mutations (Table 2). This fascinating line of research has produced some wonderful biology and biochemistry. Of special interest has been the evidence that these mutations involve differential use of fuel and enhancement of resistance to various modalities of "stress," including exposure to ultraviolet light and heat (reviewed by Martin et al. 1996). These findings are reminiscent of the longevity enhancement associated with the caloric restriction experiments in rodents discussed below.

There is no doubt that single gene variants in this organism can dramatically increase life span. As such, the findings pose a serious challenge to the "complificationists." Only recently, however, have researchers begun to quantitate the metabolic rates of these mutants. One potential scenario is that they may all exhibit decreased rates of oxygen consumption in their somatic cells. If that proves to be the case, these models of longevity may be less compelling, as they could be analogous to the longevity extension achieved in such poikilothermic organisms by the simple expediency of lowering the ambient temperature.

Single Major Genes in Fruit Flies

There have been at least three publications in recent years describing enhancement of the life spans of *Drosophila melanogaster* by simple genetic manipulations. The first involved the introduction of a gene (elongation factor 1 alpha) thought to enhance life span by increasing the efficiency of protein synthesis (Shepherd et al. 1989). The second involved the introduction of extra copies of two genes (superoxide dismutase 1 and catalase) involved in the scavenging of reactive oxygen species (Orr and Sohal 1994). The third involved the overexpression of superoxide dismutase 1 in motor neurons (Parkes et al. 1998). A difficulty with the first report was that there was no proof for the expression of the gene thought to enhance life span (a gene coding for additional expression of the elongation factor EF-1, introduced via a P element vector). The second study was given additional support by evidence that the flies were protected from oxidative damage (Sohal et al. 1995), but there remains the possibility that the results were attributable to some position effect, as not all transformed lines exhibited enhanced life spans. The third study did not consider the possibility that the strain of flies employed might have had a special propensity for late life motor neuron disease. That particular stock may have carried some private mutation or mutations that limited life span via its special vulnerability.

It can be argued that a more robust experimental design to address the question of the degree of genetic complexity of life span of fruit flies would begin with genetically heterogeneous wild type stocks, followed by indirect or direct selection of enhanced life span. Several groups, reviewed by Rose (1991), have done these experiments. The results were consistent with the predictions of the evolutionary biological theory of aging, in that they demonstrated associations with enhancement of late life fecundity with enhanced life spans. Not surprisingly, the genes influencing the emergence of long life span have been mapped to each of the major chromosomes of *Drosophila* (Luckinbill et al. 1988). While we still do not know how many genes are involved, it is already clear that life span in such wild type organisms is under polygenic controls.

Single Gene Mutations in Man

As mentioned above, some investigators consider that the gene mutation responsible for the Werner syndrome argues that a single mechanism can explain much of aging. I have argued elsewhere, however, that the Werner syndrome is best regarded as a private mutation (Martin 1997). We have much to learn about the potential role of both advantageous and disadvantageous polymorphisms at that locus, however.

The Werner syndrome (WS) is sometimes referred to as "Progeria of the Adult" to differentiate it from "Progeria of Childhood." The latter is also known as the Hutchinson-Gilford syndrome and has a number of features that differentiate it from WS, including its much earlier onset; it is most likely the result of an autosomal dominant mutation (Brown et al. 1985). WS is inherited as an autosomal recessive. Its onset is typically around the time of puberty, when there is a failure to undergo the usual adolescent growth spurt. There then follows a striking array of progeroid features, including premature graying and thinning of the hair, atrophy and altered pigmentation of the skin, regional loss of subcutaneous fat, bilateral ocular cataracts, diabetes mellitus, gonadal atrophy, osteoporosis, benign and malignant neoplasms, and a variety of forms of arteriosclerosis (atherosclerosis, arteriolosclerosis and medical calcification; Epstein et al. 1966). There are a number of phenotypic discordances with what one sees in "usual" aging, however. For example, the osteoporosis is more severe in the distal extremities than in the vertebral column. There are severe ulcerations around the Achilles heel and malleoli and, less frequently, ulcers around the elbow. These are associated with deposits of subcutaneous calcium. The neoplasms are predominantly of mesenchymal rather than epithelial origins and there is an excess of rare tumors, such as acral lentiginous melanomas (Goto et al. 1996). Somatic cells from WS subjects undergo accelerated rates of replicative senescence (Martin et al. 1970). There are reasons to suspect, however, that the mechanism whereby these cells exit the cell cycle may be different from that which obtains in cells from normal individuals. There are three lines of evidence to support this assertion. First, there is the observation that the *cFOS* gene can be readily induced in senescent WS cells (Oshima et al. 1995). Second, while there appears to be an accelerated loss of telomere restriction fragments in serially passaged WS cells, these appear to be significantly longer than comparably senescent cells from controls (Schulz et al. 1996). Thus, loss of telomere repeats may not be the reason that WS cells undergo replicative senescence. Third, WS somatic cells exhibit elongated S phases and some cells appear to become arrested in S (Poot et al. 1992). There are several lines of evidence indicating that WS cells are prone to chromosomal and intragenic mutations, particularly deletions (references cited in Martin 1997). Thus, some might argue that, even if the WS mutation results in a caricature of aging, it could provide a line of important evidence supporting an important role of genomic instability in the genesis of senescent phenotypes. There are, of course, numerous other genes that can modulate genomic stability. Mutations and polymorphisms at such loci may thus be important contributors to a polygenic basis for senescence.

The WS locus (*WRN*) was cloned in 1996 (Yu et al. 1996). Since that time, numerous independent mutations have been documented (Oshima et al. 1996; Yu et al. 1997). All result in truncated products of a protein that is a member of the *RecQ* class of helicases. Biochemical experiments have established that the protein indeed functions to unwind double stranded DNA (Suzuki et al. 1997; Gray et al. 1997). The gene product is therefore likely to be of importance in one or more key transactions involving DNA (replication, recombination, repair, transcription, and chromosome segregation). It is thus not surprising that the cells exhibit a mutator phenotype and that the patients are prone to develop cancer. The discovery that a helicase gene is associated with premature atherosclerosis is surprising, however, and supports the pioneering work of the late Earl P. Benditt implicating somatic mutation or viral transformation in the etiology of atheromas (Benditt and Benditt 1973). It is now important to ask if more subtle alteration of the gene product ("leaky" mutations, polymorphisms) might play a role in susceptibility to atherogenesis. An initial report of an association with a polymorphism with susceptibility to myocardial infarction in a Japanese population supports such a role (Ye et al. 1997). Another question of public health significance is the extent to which heterozygous carriers of mutations at *WRN* might predispose individuals to age-associated diseases. Such a connection is supported by evidence that somatic cells from such subjects exhibit a degree of sensitivity to a genotoxic agent (4-nitroquinoline-1-oxide) that is intermediate to that exhibited by wild type and homozygous mutant cells from members of the same pedigree (Ogburn et al. 1997). While there is no obvious clinical evidence that heterozygotes suffer premature debilities, there is some evidence from family studies that they may be at increased risk for neoplasia (Goto et al. 1981).

Caloric Restriction in Rodents

One of the most reproducible findings in gerontology is the enhancement of the life span of rodents by the simple expediency of reducing calories in an otherwise nutritionally sufficient diet (reviewed by Masoro 1996). The fact that a single environmental manipulation (input of calories) can delay multiple diseases and extend life span argues against a plethora of mechanisms of aging. Unlike the situation in nematodes, mammalian biologists believe they have ruled out a role for decreased metabolic rate as an explanation for these findings (Masoro 1996). The findings are consistent with some general up-regulation of defenses against a variety of endogenous and exogenous stressors, including oxidative stress. There is indeed considerable evidence that resistance to such stressors may underlie gene action in the determination of life span for a wide variety of organisms (Martin et al. 1996). Thus, allelic variation of a large number of loci relevant to such gene action could modulate rates of aging and susceptibility to senescent phenotypes, consistent with a polygenic basis for aging as it unfolds in genetically heterogeneous species, such as *Homo sapiens*. It remains to be seen, of course, if caloric restriction influences the life span of higher primates.

Conclusions

Taken as a whole, and with particular emphasis upon aging in man, we can conclude that aging and age-related diseases are under highly polygenic controls. The author thus favors the "complificationist" view. The fact that the extensions of life span by single gene mutations in *C. elegans* and by caloric restriction in mammals appear to involve alternative pathways of fuel utilization, however, suggests that the polygenes are acting within a small number of metabolic pathways under control of a smaller subset of genes, thus encouraging more research by the "simplificationists."

References

Austad SN (1993) Retarded senescence in an insular population of Virginia possums (Didelphis virginiana). J Zool Lond 229:695–708

Austad SN (1997) Why we age: what science is discovering about the body's journey through life. John Wiley & Sons, New York

Benditt EP, Benditt JM (1973) Evidence for a monoclonal origin of human atherosclerotic plaques. Proc Natl Acad Sci (USA) 70:1753–1756

Blacker D, Tanzi RE (1998) The genetics of Alzheimer disease: current status and future prospects. Arch Neurol 55:294–296

Brown WT, Kieras FJ, Houck GE, Jr, Dutkowski R, Jenkins EC (1985) A comparison of adult and childhood progerias: Werner syndrome and Hutchinson-Gilford progeria syndrome. Adv Exp Med Biol 190:229–244

Brown J, Ashworth A, Gydesen S, Sorensen A, Rossor M, Hardy J, Collinge J (1995) Familial nonspecific dementia maps to chromosome 3. Human Mol Genet 4:1625–1628

Bullido MJ, Artiga MJ, Recuero M, Sastre I, Garcia MA, Aldudo J, Lendon C, Han SW, Morris IC, Frank A, Vazquez J, Goate A, Valdivieso F (1998) A polymorphism in the regulatory region of APOE associated with risk for Alzheimer's dementia. Nat Genet 18:69–71

Corder EH, Saunders AM, Strittmatter WJ, Schmechel DE, Gaskell PC, Small GW, Roses AD, Haines JL, Pericak-Vance MA (1993) Gene dose of apolipoprotein E type 4 allele and the risk of Alzheimer's disease in late onset families. Science 261:921–923

Ebert RH, 2nd, Shammas MA, Sohal BH, Sohal RS, Egilmez NK, Ruggles S, Shmookler Reis RJ (1996) Defining genes that govern longevity in *Caenorhabditis elegans*. Dev Genet 18:131–43

Epstein CJ, Martin GM, Schultz AL, Motulsky AG (1966) Werner's syndrome a review of its symptomatology, natural history, pathologic features, genetics and relationships to the natural aging process. Medicine 45:177–221

Evans DA, Funkenstein HH, Albert MS, Scherr PA, Cook NR, Chown MJ, Herbert LE, Hennekens CH, Taylor JO, (1989) Prevalence of Alzheimer's disease in a community population of older persons. Higher than previously reported. JAMA 262:2551–2556

Ewbank JJ, Barnes TM, Lakowski B, Lussier M, Bussey H, Hekimi S (1997) Structural and functional conservation of the *Caenorhabditis elegans* timing gene clk-1. Science 275:980–983

Friedman DB, Johnson TE (1988) A mutation in the age-1 gene in *Caenorhabditis elegans* lengthens life and reduces hermaphrodite fertility. Genetics 118:75–86

Gerdes LU, Klausen IC, Sihm I, Faergeman O (1992) Apolipoprotein E polymorphism in a Danish population compared to findings in 45 other study populations around the world. Genet Epidemiol 9:155–167

Goate A, Chartier-Harlin MC, Mullan M, Brown J, Crawford F, Fidani L, Giuffra L, Haynes A, Irving N, James L, Mant R, Newton P, Rooke K, Roques P, Talbot C, Pericak-Vance M, Roses A, Williamson R, Rossor M, Owen M, Hardy J (1991) Segregation of a missense mutation in the amyloid precursor protein gene with familial Alzheimer's disease. Nature 349:704–706

G'omez-Isla T, Price JL, McKeel DW, Jr., Morris JC, Growdon JH, Hyman BT (1996) Profound loss of layer II entorhinal cortex neurons occurs in very mild Alzheimer's disease. J Neurosci 16:4491–4500

Goto M, Tanimoto K, Horiuchi Y, Sasazuki T (1981) Family analysis of Werner's syndrome: a survey of 42 Japanese families with a review of the literature. Clin Genet 19:8–15

Goto M, Miller RW, Ishikawa Y, Sugano H (1996) Excess of rare cancers in Werner syndrome (adult progeria). Cancer Epidemiol Biomarkers Prev 5:239–246

Gray MD, Shen JC, Kamath-Loeb AS, Blank A, Sopher BL, Martin GM, Oshima J, Loeb LA (1997) The Werner syndrome protein is a DNA helicase. Nat Genet 17:100–103

Hutton M, Hardy J (1997) The presenilins and Alzheimer's disease. Human Mol Genet 6:1639–1646

Hutton M, Lendon CL, Rizzu P, Baker M, Froelich S, Houlden H, Pickering-Brown S, Chakraverty S, Isaacs A, Grover A, Hackett J, Adamson J, Lincoln S, Dickson D, Davies P, Petersen RC, Stevens M, de Graaff E, Wauters E, van Baren J, Hillebrand M, Joosse M, Kwon JM, Nowotny P, Che LK, Norton J, Morris JC, Reed LA, Trojanowski J, Basun H, Lannfelt L, Neystat M, Fahn S, Dark F, Tannenberg T, Dodd PR, Hayward N, Kwok JBJ, Schofield PR, Andreadis A, Snowden J, Craufurd D, Neary D, Owen F, Oostra BA, Hardy J, Goate A, van Swieten J, Mann D, Lynch T, Heutink P (1998) Association of missense and 5'-splice-site mutations in tau with the inherited dementia FTDP-17. Nature 393:702–705

Johnson TE, Wood WB (1982) Genetic analysis of *Caenorhabditis elegans*. Proc Natl Acad Sci (USA) 79:6603–6607

Joutel A, Corpechot C, Ducros A, Vahedi K, Chabriat H, Mouton P, Alamowitsch S, Domenga V, Cecillion M, Marechal E, Maciazek J, Vayssiere C, Cruaud C, Cabanis EA, Ruchoux MM, Weissenbach J, Bach JF, Bousser MG, Tournier-Lasserve E (1996) Notch3 mutations in CADASIL, a hereditary adult-onset condition causing stroke and dementia. Nature 383:707–710

Kenyon C, Chang J, Gensch E, Rudner A, Tabtiang R (1993) A *C. elegans* mutant that lives twice as long as wild type. Nature 366:461–464

Kimura KD, Tissenbaum HA, Liu Y, Ruvkun G (1997) Daf-2, an insulin receptor-like gene that regulates longevity and diapause in *Caenorhabditis elegans*. Science 277:942–946

Levy-Lahad E, Wasco W, Poorkaj P, Romano DM, Oshima J, Pettingell WH, Yu CE, Jondro PD, Schmidt SD, Wang K, Crowley AC, Fu YH, Guenette SY, Galas D, Nemens E, Wijsman EM, Bird TD, Schellenberg GD, Tanzi RE (1995) Candidate gene for the chromosome 1 familial Alzheimer's disease locus. Science 269:973–977

Luckinbill LS, Clare MJ (1985) Selection for life span in *Drosophila melanogaster*. Heredity 55:9–18

Luckinbill LS, Clare MJ (1987) Successful selection for increased longevity in *Drosophila*: analysis of the survival data and presentation of a hypothesis on the genetic regulation of longevity. Exp Gerontol 22:221–226

Luckinbill LS, Graves JL, Reed AH, Koetsawang S (1988) Localizing genes that defer senescence in *Drosophila melanogaster*. Heredity 60:367–374

Martin GM (1978) Genetic syndromes in man with potential relevance to the pathobiology of aging. Birth Defects Orig Artic Ser 14:5–39

Martin GM (1997) The Werner mutation: does it lead to a "public" or "private" mechanism of aging? Mol Med 3:356–358

Martin GM, Sprague CA, Epstein CJ (1970) Replicative life-span of cultivated human cells. Effects of donor's age, tissue, and genotype. Lab Invest 23:86–92

Martin GM, Austad SN, Johnson TE (1996) Genetic analysis of ageing: role of oxidative damage and environmental stresses. Nat Genet 13:25–34

Masoro EJ (1996) Possible mechanisms underlying the antiaging actions of caloric restriction. Toxicol Pathol 24:738–741

Medawar PB (1952) An unsolved problem of biology. HK Lewis, London

Morris JZ, Tissenbaum HA, Ruvkun G (1996) A phosphatidylinositol-3-OH kinase family member regulating longevity and diapause in *Caenorhabitis elegans*. Nature 382:536–539

Ogburn CE, Oshima J, Poot M, Chen R, Hunt KE, Gollahon KA, Rabinovitch PS, Martin GM (1997) An apoptosis-inducing genotoxin differentiates heterozygotic carriers for Werner helicase mutations from wild-type and homozygous mutants. Hum Genet 101:121–125

Orr WC, Sohal RS (1994) Extension of life-span by overexpression of superoxide dismutase and catalase in *Drosophila melanogaster*. Science 263:1128–1130

Oshima J, Campisi J, Tannock TC, Martin GM (1995) Regulation of c-fos expression in senescing Werner syndrome fibroblasts differs from that observed in senescing fibroblasts from normal donors. J Cell Physiol 162:277–283

Oshima J, Yu CE, Piussan C, Klein G, Jabkowski J, Balci S, Miki T, Nakura J, Ogihara T, Ells J, Smith M, Melaragno MI, Fraccaro M, Scappaticci S, Matthews J, Ouais S, Jarzebowicz A, Schellenberg GD, (1996) Homozygous and compound heterozygous mutations at the Werner syndrome locus. Human Mol Genet 5:1909–1913

Parkes TL, Elia AJ, Dickinson D, Hilliker AJ, Phillips JP, Gabrielle LB (1998) Extension of *Drosophila* life, span by overexpression of human SOD1 in motorneurons. Nat Genet 19:171–174

Pericak-Vance MA, Bass MP, Yamaoka LH, Gaskell PC, Scott WK, Terwedow HA, Menold MM, Conneally PM, Small GW, Vance JM, Saunders AM, Roses AD, Haines JL (1997) Complete genomic screen in late-onset familial Alzheimer disease: evidence for a new locus on chromosome 12. JAMA 278:1237–1241

Poorkaj P, Bird TD, Wijsman E, Nemens E, Garruto RM, Anderson L, Andreadis A, Wiederholt WC, Raskind M, Schellenberg GD (1998) Tau is a candidate gene for chromosome 17 frontotemporal dementia. Ann Neurol 43:815–825

Poot M, Hoehn H, Runger TM, Martin GM (1992) Impaired S-phase transit of Werner syndrome cells expressed in lymphoblastoid cell lines. Exp Cell Res 202:267–273

Rose MR (1991) Evolutionary biology of aging. Oxford University Press, New York

Rose MR, Charlesworth B (1981) Genetics of life history in *Drosophila melanogaster*. II. Exploratory selection experiments. Genetics 97:187–196

Rose MR, Graves JL Jr (1989) What evolutionary biology can do for gerontology. J Gerontol 44:B27–29

Schulz VP, Zakian VA, Ogburn CE, MyKay J, Jarzebowicz AA, Edland SD, Martin GM (1996) Accelerated loss of telomeric repeats may not explain accelerated replicative decline of Werner syndrome cells. Human Genet 97:750–754

Shepherd JC, Walldorf U, Hug P, Gehring WJ (1989) Fruit flies with additional expression of the elongation factor EF-1 alpha live longer. Proc Natl Acad Sci (USA) 86:7520–7521

Sherrington R, Rogaev EI, Liang Y, Rogaeva EA, Levesque G, Ikeda M, Chi H, Lin C, Li G, Holman K, Tsuda T, Mar L, Foncin JF, Bruni AC, Montesi MP, Sorbi S, Rainero I, Pinessi L, Nee L, Chumakov I, Pollen D, Brookes A, Sanseau P, Polinsky RJ, Wasco W, Da Silva HAR, Haines JL, Pericak-Vance MA, Tanzi RE, Roses AD, Fraser PE, Rommens JM, St. George-Hyslop PH, Ikegami H, Higaki J, Edland SD, Martin GM, Ogihara T (1995) Cloning of a gene bearing missense mutations in early-onset familial Alzheimer's disease. Nature 375:754–760

Sohal RS, Agarwal A, Agarwal S, Orr WC (1995) Simultaneous overexpression of copper- and zinc-containing superoxide dismutase and catalase retards age-related oxidative damage and increases metabolic potential in *Drosophila melanogaster*. J Biol Chem 270:15671–15674

Suzuki N, Shimamoto A, Imamura O, Kuromitsu J, Kitao S, Goto M, Furnichi Y, Ikegami H, Higaki J, Edland SD, Martin GM, Ogihara T (1997) DNA helicase activity in Werner's syndrome gene product synthesized in a baculovirus system. Nucleic Acids Res 25:2973–2978

Van Voorhies WA (1992) Production of sperm reduces nematode lifespan. Nature 360:456–458

Varkey JP, Muhlrad PJ, Minniti AN, Do B, Ward S (1995) The *Caenorhabditis elegans* spe-26 gene is necessary to form spermatids and encodes a protein similar to the actin-associated proteins kelch and scruin. Genes Dev 9:1074–1086

Ye L, Miki T, Nakura J, Oshima J, Kamino K, Rakugi H, Ikegami H, Higaki J, Edland SD, Martin GM, Ogihara T (1997) Association of a polymorphic variant of the Werner helicase gene with myocardial infarction in a Japanese population. Am J Med Genet 68:494–498

Yu CE, Oshima J, Fu YH, Wijsman EM, Hisama F, Alisch R, Matthews S, Nakura J, Miki T, Ovais S, Martin GM, Mulligan J, Schellenberg GD (1996) Positional cloning of the Werner's syndrome gene. Science 272:258–262

Yu CE, Oshima J, Wijsman EM, Nakura J, Miki T, Piussan C, Matthews S, Fu YH, Mulligan J, Martin GM, Schellenberg GD (1997) Mutations in the consensus helicase domains of the Werner syndrome gene. Am J Hum Genet 60:330–341

Zwaan B, Bulsma R, Hoekstra RF (1995) Direct selection on life in *Drosophila melanogaster*. Evolution 49:649–659

How Mediterranean Fruit Flies
Resist Aging, Live Long and Remain Fertile

J. R. Carey[1]

Introduction

The Mediterranean fruit fly (*Ceratitis capitata*; medfly) is one of the most successful insects in the world with respect to its ability to invade new regions (Carey 1991). The species has spread from its origins in tropical Africa to virtually all areas of Mediterranean Europe, North Africa, and the Middle East, to most countries in South and Central America, to isolated pockets in North America (e. g., California and Florida), and to several regions in the Pacific, including the Hawaiian Islands and western Australia (Carey 1997).

One reason for the medfly's invasion success is that it is capable of persisting in small, sparsely distributed populations when hosts, food and mates are scarce. For example, entomologists frequently report the presence of extremely small medfly populations in regions where annual re-invasion is unlikely, including remote areas of Israel (Rivnay 1950), Hawaii (Vargas et al. 1983), California (Carey 1996), Australia (Maelzer 1990) and Greece (Papadopoulos et al. 1996). Inasmuch as these remote areas lack larval hosts for much of the year and medfly preadults (eggs-to-pupae) are not capable of diapause (Christenson and Foote 1960), one of the most important physiological adaptations that allow the medfly to persist at low population levels is the ability of the adult females to bridge unfavorable periods by reducing their rate of aging. Despite the importance of understanding how medflies survive in isolated regions with few resources, surprisingly few studies have been conducted on the physiological ecology of this species. And virtually no research has been published on the ecological context of aging in wild populations.

The underlying motive for this paper stems from the recent finding from laboratory studies in which medfly females were found to live longer and be capable of reproducing at later ages if they were maintained on a sugar-only diet at younger ages and then switched to a full diet at older ages (Carey et al., 1998). These findings are important because they suggest that there may be two physiological modes of aging – a waiting mode in which reproduction is low and survival high, and a reproductive mode in which reproduction and survival are both high initially but decrease rapidly at older ages. This concept more securely links the

[1] Department of Entomology, University of California, Davis, CA 95616-8584, USA.

J.-M. Robine et al. (Eds.)
Research and Perspectives in Longevity
The Paradoxes of Longevity
© Springer-Verlag Berlin Heidelberg New York 1999

aging literature (Finch 1991) with the physiological ecology literature concerned with the response of animals to periods of host, mate, and/or food shortages.

Baseline Medfly life Table Studies

The starting point for investigations on medfly aging was publication of the paper by Carey et al. (1992) reporting the results of the large-scale life table study of Mediterranean fruit flies (*Ceratitis capitata*). Age-specific mortality was monitored in 1.2 million medflies over their lifetimes at the Moscamed fruit fly rearing facility in Tapachula, Mexico. The main finding from this study was that death rates slowed at older ages, which implied that senescence cannot be characterized as an ever-increasing risk of death, that the Gompertz mortality model did not describe a unitary pattern or mortality at older ages in all species, and that there was no absolute life span limit.

A subtle feature of the mortality curve presented in this original paper, but one that was not addressed in it, was the appearance of a mortality "shoulder" (Fig. 1). The follow-up analysis of the data on the sex-specific mortality patterns (Carey et al. 1995 a), as well as a separate study on the effects of density on the

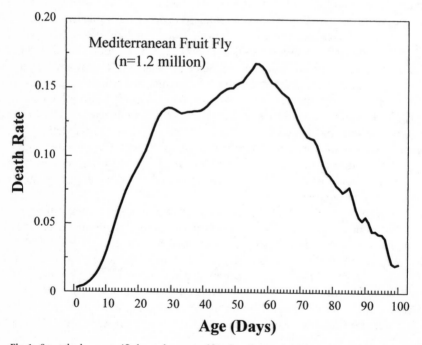

Fig. 1. Smoothed age-specific hazard rates medflies based on an initial number of 1.2 million individuals (both sexes). Note presence of the mortality "shoulder" at about 3 weeks (redrawn from Carey et al. 1992)

mortality patterns at older ages (Carey et al. 1995 b), revealed that this "shoulder" was expressed in female cohorts but not in male cohorts. The implication of this observation was that changes at the level of the individual (i.e., reproductive physiology) may account for changes in mortality trajectories at the level of the cohort.

This hypothesis, that individual-level changes in reproductive physiology explain the surge in mortality at younger ages in female cohorts, was tested by Müller et al. (1997). Experiments were conducted on medfly cohorts totaling over 400,000 flies maintained on one of two dietary regimes: 1) a sugar-plus protein diet in which flies were provided with sucrose and a protein source (referred to as a "full diet"); and 2) a protein-free diet in which flies were provided with a diet consisting only of sugar (protein-deprived). The main results from this study included: 1) life expectancy at eclosion was reduced in both male and female medflies if they were deprived of protein, though this reduction was greater in females (16.5 vs 12.1 days) than in males (15.2 vs 14.3 days); and 2) the sex differential in life expectancy favors females when cohorts are maintained on a full diet but reverses when flies are maintained on a sugar-only diet. As shown in Figure 2, the reversal of the male-female life expectancy differential is caused by a sustained surge in early female mortality under protein deprivation that is tied to egg-laying and physiological processes.

The finding that the surge in mortality at younger ages in sugar-fed female cohorts accounts for the significant difference in life expectancy between sugar-fed and protein-fed females, as well as for the reversal in sex-specific life expec-

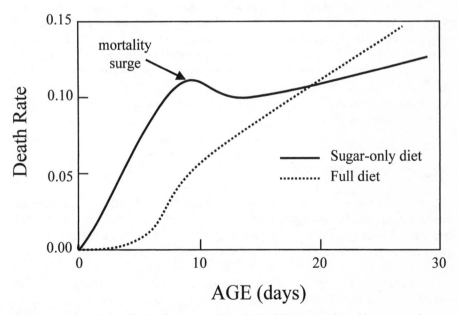

Fig. 2. Death rates for medfly females (n = 30,000 individuals) maintained on either sugar-only or a full diet (redrawn from Müller et al. 1997)

tancy, provides support for the initial hypothesis that individual-level changes in the reproductive physiology account for the mortality "shoulder" in female cohorts. This finding foreshadows the more recent discovery suggesting that medflies increase their survival rates by switching to a "waiting" mode of reproduction. In other words, the followup study by Müller et al. (1997) and a more recent one by Carey et al. (1998) suggest that the shoulder in the hazard curse of the original life table study of 1.2 million medflies (Carey et al. 1992), as well as the decline in mortality at the oldest ages, may be partly explained as due to the sugar-only diet on which the flies were maintained – the dietary regime caused the flies to remain in the "waiting" mode throughout their lives.

How Medflies Live Long and Remain Fertile

The ability of insects such as the medfly to enter arrested states and thus prolong survival and still retain the ability to reproduce evolved as an adaptation to synchronize the life cycle of animals with the rhythm of the environment and to insure that the active stages are present when conditions become favorable for reproduction (Andrewartha and Birch 1954; Mansingh 1971). Danks (1987) classified arrested states of animals as one of two types: 1) *predictive*, which refers to dormancy initiated in advance of the adverse conditions, such as hibernation in mammals or diapause in overwintering insects. In this case the conditions are variable but predictable; and 2) *consequential*, which is initiated in response to the adverse conditions themselves (e.g. germination of many plant seeds). This type of dormancy in animals is expected to evolve in environments that are unpredictable. In the following sections I describe and present data that reveal three ways in which medflies postpone their rate of aging as a *consequential* response to their environment: 1) by remaining a virgin – a consequence of not finding a mate; 2) by retaining matured eggs – a consequence of not having access to ovipositional hosts; and 3) by not manufacturing eggs – a consequence of not finding a source of dietary protein.

Virginity Prolongs Life

Many studies have documented the greater longevity of virgins over non-virgins, including studies on *Drosophila* (Smith 1958; Fowler and Partridge 1989; Partridge and Andrews 1985; Partridge 1986), the housefly, *Musca domestica* (Ragland and Sohal 1973), and the bruchiid beetle *Callosobruchus maculatus* (Tatar et al. 1993). To verify that this general principle also holds for medflies, we conducted large-scale life table studies on this species by gathering mortality data on 35,000 females maintained in all-female (virgin) cages and on 30,000 females maintained in mixed-sex (non-virgin) cages and fed a sugar-only diet (P. Liedo and J. R. Carey, unpublished data).

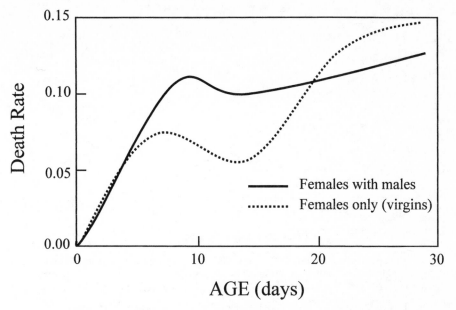

Fig. 3. Death rates of female medflies maintained in all-female (i. e., virgin) or mixed sex cages. Curves were computed using mortality data on 35,000 and 30,000 individuals for virgin and non-virgin cages, respectively (unpublished data from P. Liedo and J. Carey)

The result of these studies revealed that the life expectancy of females maintained in same-sex cages exceeded the life expectancy of females maintained in mixed-sex cages by 1.3 days (14.7 vs 16.1 days). This life expectancy differential was due to differences in mortality rates at younger ages. These rates reveal that death rates were approximately the same between virgin and non-virgin females for the first 5 days, at which time they diverged until the flies were nearly 3 weeks of age (Fig. 3). At this time the death rates for females in same-sex cages crossed over and exceeded the death rates for females maintained in mixed-sex cages. In general, the finding that the life expectancy at eclosion of unmated medfly females is greater than the life expectancy of mated females is consistent with the findings in virtually all other life table studies on virginity in insects (Reznick 1985; Bell and Koufopanou 1986).

Delayed or Intermittent Egg Laying Reduces Aging Rate

It is widely known that medflies often encounter periods when suitable hosts for oviposition are unavailable, ranging from a few days for an individual fly to find a scarce host to several months for entire populations to site and wait while hosts disappear and reappear due to seasonal changes (Drew et al. 1983; Fletcher et al. 1978; Meats and Khoo 1976). Because little is known about the demographic response of medflies to discontinuities in host availability, Carey et al. (1986)

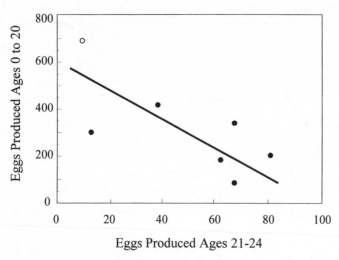

Fig. 4. Relationship between total reproduction during the first 20 days and reproduction from days 21 to 24 in medfly cohorts subjected to various host deprivation regimes. Open circle denotes control cohort in which females had access to hosts *ad libitum* (data from Table 2 in Carey et al. 1986)

conducted studies in which daily reproduction and survival were measured in cohorts of medflies subjected to periods of host deprivation. The design concept for this study was that two conditions were necessary to completely specify a period of host deprivation: 1) *level*, defined as the percentage of the total days in which the host is absent over a specified period; and 2) *pattern*, defined as the sequence of host days and host-free days over a specified period. The number of eggs produced by experimental females that had access to hosts early in the number produced by the 24 days of the study (control flies) was far fewer in the last 4 days than, females that were deprived of hosts at younger ages. For example, the control flies produced an average of 680 eggs/female during the first 20 days of the experiment but only 9.7 eggs/female in the last 4 days. By contrast, flies that were deprived of hosts for the first 16 days produced an average of 67 eggs/female during the last 4 days or around 6-fold more eggs than did the control flies. Overall the flies that were host-deprived at younger ages were capable of producing more eggs/day at older ages than were flies that had been laying throughout their lives, irrespective of the level and/or pattern of host deprivation. The number of eggs that were laid at early ages was inversely related to the number of eggs laid at older ages (Fig. 4) and directly related to total mortality after 24 days (Fig. 5). In general, the host deprivation study by Carey et al. (1986) revealed that: 1) medfly egg production is not only affected by a female's chronological age but also by her previous reproductive effort; and 2) although the cause of medfly egg production levels can be qualitatively separated into age effects and reproductive effects, no simply quantitative relationship exists between these two factors. In other words, it is not possible to assign a unit cost to future reproduction. Although a reproductive pacemaker may exist – individ-

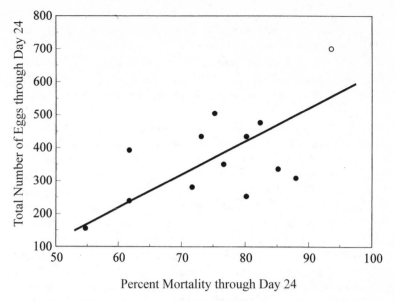

Fig. 5. Relationship between egg production in medfly cohorts subjected to various host deprivation regimes for 24 days and percentage mortality at the end of this period. Open circle denotes control cohorts in which females had access to hosts *ad libitum* (data from Tables 1 and 4 in Carey et al. 1986)

ual medfly females may only be endowed with a fixed number of germinal egg cells determined partly by genetics, partly by the environment and partly by chance – there are clearly other factors besides current and total reproductive output that determine longevity.

Protein Deprivation Suppresses Egg Production and Prolongs Life

Courtice and Drew (1984) studied the nutritional ecology of two fruit fly relatives of the medfly in Australia and concluded that "... food supply for egg production is the factor primarily responsible for fluctuations in numbers of *Dacus tryoni* and *D. neohumeralis*, the two major pest species in eastern Australia." Drew et al. (1983) stated "Our work suggests that nutrition, and particularly adult nutrition, is of overriding importance to the activity and numbers of fruit flies."

These findings provide context for the recent findings concerning dietary restriction of adult females by Carey et al. (1998), who concluded that the life history of medflies can be characterized by two physiological modes with different demographic schedules of fertility and survival: 1) a waiting mode, in which both mortality and reproduction are low; and 2) a reproductive mode, in which mortality is very low at the onset of egg laying but accelerates as eggs are laid. This discovery was the result of an experiment in which an initial pool of 2,500 adults of each sex was maintained in single pair cages with sugar and water and subgroups of 100 pairs were selected at 30, 60 and 90 days, provided with a full diet *ad libitum* and their reproduction and survival monitored until the last female died. Lifetime reproduction and survival were also monitored from eclosion in two 100-pair control cohorts – one on sugar-only and the other on a full diet. The following specific results point to this two-mode aging system: 1) the life expectancy of flies in all three treatments increased immediately on the days when they were given a full diet after having been maintained on a sugar-only diet; 2) the life expectancy of the full-diet control flies at eclosion was not only similar to the life expectancy of the treatment flies at the ages when they were first given a full diet, but also similar to their life expectancies 30 and 60 days after they were first given full diet, even though their absolute ages differed substantially; 3) the duration of the life-expectancy advantage in medflies maintained on a full diet was short relative to that of medflies maintained on a sugar-only diet. This general response of a short-term gain but a long-term reduction in life expectancy for flies switched from sugar to a full diet was evidenced in all three treatment cohorts; 4) female medflies maintained on a sugar-only diet and then switched to a full diet were capable of producing eggs at all ages tested, but lifetime egg production decreased as the age at the time of switch increased; 5) age-specific death rates for three of the 100-fly cohorts revealed striking similarities in their trajectories after they were given access to a full diet, even though their chronological ages differed by up to two months. They shifted to a different mortality "track" once their diet was switched from sugar to full and they began laying eggs.

The discovery that medflies experience two separate modes of aging is fundamental to biological, evolutionary and ecological research on aging because it provides a basis for replacing the unrealistic assumption of fixed demographic schedules in the Lotka equation, which is used as the basis for the evolutionary theory of aging, with the more realistic assumption that these schedules can be induced and thus are highly plastic. Research on the nature of the induced physiological shift that occurs when medflies are switched to protein may open a window into the fundamental processes that determine longevity (see Vaupel et al. 1998).

Discussion

Medflies are able to retain their youth at older ages when conditions are unfavorable for reproduction by remaining young physiologically even though they are old chronologically. Thus one of the demographic consequences of postponed aging is that chronological age becomes less relevant to the concepts of longevity and life span than does physiological age. Whereas physical (chronological) time is measured in hours, days, and years and is assumed to flow evenly and inexorably at the rate of solar time, physiological time does not pass at a constant rate through the time frame of physical time. Thus the more development that accumulates between two calendar dates, the faster time may be said to pass for the developing insect. Or, for sexually mature adults, the more eggs that are matured and deposited between two points in time, the more rapidly the insect may be said to age (Carrel 1931). An insect in the egg stage cannot become an adult without first passing through the larval and pupal stages although the stages through which it passes are, of course, independent of the development rate. Thus the direction and sequence of this development process is deterministic and it is most appropriately tracked on a physiological rather than on a chronological time scale.

The data on postponed aging in the medfly suggest that it may be useful to view insect aging and reproduction in the context of a physiological rather than a chronological time scale. Whereas the conventional Lexis diagram (Pressat 1985) consists of a series of life-lines representing individuals increasing in age in direct proportion to the increase in calender time, a modified life-line that follows a physiological time scale when an individual enters an arrested state will appear warped. The contrast between the two life-lines is shown in Figure 6 where the left-most linear curve depicts chronological age increasing at exactly the same rate as physical time but the right-most non-linear curve depicts physiological age changing at different rates relative to physical time. This schematic

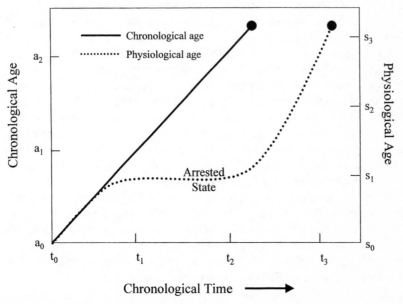

Fig. 6. Lexis diagram showing: 1) the conventional life line depicting the exact relationship between physical (calendar) time and chronological age – an organism's chronological age increases at the same rate as physical time. Chronological age, denoted a_i, passes at the same rate as physical time, denoted t_i; and 2) a physiological age life line where biological age is a non-linear function of chronological time. Physiological age/stage, denoted s_i, accumulates at different rates relative to physical time. An organism may enter an arrested state when conditions are unfavorable for growth or reproduction and thus its developmental and/or reproductive rate warps relative to its chronological age scale

illustrates why two individuals experiencing different environments – one where females enter an arrested stage and the other environment where females actively reproduce – will age at drastically different rates relative to chronological time.

The concept of physiological aging interpreted in a biogerontological context has several important implications with respect to aging and longevity. First, it renders invalid the concept of a fixed maximal age. This is because, unlike the chronological age of an individual, which progresses according to calendar time, the physiological age of an individual progresses according to the interaction between its physiological predisposition and its environment. Thus different conditions of host, food and mate availability will yield different physiological aging rates and thus different chronological life spans and maximal ages.

Second, up to now the evolutionary biology of aging was based on the unrealistic assumption that demographic schedules are fixed. The discovery that medflies experience two separate modes of aging is fundamental to biological, evolutionary and ecological research on aging because it provides a basis for replacing the former unrealistic assumption with the more realistic assumption that these schedules can be induced and thus are highly plastic. Thus research on the nature of the induced physiological shift that occurs when medflies are switched to protein may open a window into the fundamental processes that determine longevity. That demographic schedules can be induced will provide the empirical groundwork to stimulate development of a whole new class of demographic concepts, particularly those that assume that longevity is mediated through reproduction, which, in turn, is linked to the environment. Models that capture the interplay of birth and death rather than assume that these vital rates are independent will have a profound impact on the development of new theories of aging, as well as serve as touchstones for the emerging area of biodemography (see Carey and Gruenfelder 1997; Wachter and Finch 1997).

Third, by viewing the waiting mode of reproduction in the context of dormancy, postponed aging can be situated on one end of a dormancy continuum ranging from quiescence, reproductive diapause and shallow torpor to hibernation, aestivation and cryptobiosis on the other. Waiting strategies for prolonging survival while maintaining reproductive potential have been extensively documented in the physiological, ecological and natural history literature. The genes that regulate the transition to the waiting mode and survival in this mode are closely linked to longevity in nematode worms and yeast (Jazwinski 1996; Finch and Tanzi 1997). Thus research on the waiting mode and transitions in and out of it may provide key insights for understanding how many species remain young and retain their ability to reproduce at older ages in the wild.

References

Andrewartha HG, Birch LC (1954) The distribution and abundance of animals. The University of Chicago Press, Chicago

Bell G, Koufopanou V (1986) The cost of reproduction, In: Dawkins R, Ridley M (eds) Oxford surveys in evolutionary biology. Oxford University Press, New York, pp. 83–131

Carey JR (1991) Establishment of the Mediterranean fruit fly in California. Science 253:1369–1373

Carey JR (1996) The incipient Mediterranean fruit fly population in California: implications for invasion biology. Ecology 77:1690–1697

Carey JR (1997) The future of the Mediterranean fruit fly population in California: a predictive framework. Biol Conserv 78:35–50

Carey JR, Gruenfelder C (1997) Population biology of the elderly. In: Wachter K, Finch, C. (eds) Between Zeus and the salmon: the biodemography of longevity. National Academy Press, Washington, DC

Carey JR, Krainacker D, Vargas R (1986) Life history response of Mediterranean fruit fly females to periods of host deprivation. Entomologia experimentalis et applicata 42:159–167

Carey JR, Liedo P, Orozco D, Vaupel JW (1992) Slowing of mortality rates at older ages in large medfly cohorts. Science 258:457–461

Carey JR, Liedo P, Orozco D, Tatar M, Vaupel JW (1995 a). A male-female longevity paradox in medfly cohorts. J Anim Ecol 64:107–116

Carey JR, Liedo P, Vaupel JW (1995 b) Mortality dynamics of density in the Mediterranean fruit fly. Exp Gerontol 30:605–629

Carey JR, Liedo P, Müller H-G, Wang J-L and Vaupel JW (1998) Dual modes of aging in Mediterranean fruit fly females. Science 281: 396–398

Carrel A (1931) Physiological time. Science 74:618–621

Christenson LD, Foote RH (1960) Biology of fruit flies. Ann Rev Entomol 5:171–192

Courtice AC, Drew RAI (1984) Bacterial regulation of abundance in tropical fruit flies (Diptera: Tephritidae). Aust Zool 21:251–268

Danks HV (1987) Insect dormancy: an ecological perspective. Biol Survey Can Mono Series No. 1

Drew RAI Courtice AC, Teakle DS (1983) Bacteria as a natural source of food for adult fruit flies (Diptera: Tephritidae). Oecologia 60:279–284

Finch C (1991) Longevity, senescence and the genome. University of Chicago Press, Chicago

Finch CE, (1997) Comparative perspectives on plasticity in human aging and life spans. In: Wachter K, Finch C (eds) Between Zeus and the salmon: the biodemography of longevity. National Academy Press, Washington DC, pp. 245–268

Finch CE, Tanzi RE (1997). Genetics of aging. Science 278:407–411

Fletcher BS, Pappas S, Kapatos E (1978) Changes in the ovaries of olive flies (*Dacus oleae* (Gmelin)) during the summer, and their relationship to temperature, humidity and fruit availability. Ecol Entomol 3:99–107

Fowler K, Partridge L (1989) A cost of mating in female fruit flies. Nature 338:760–761

Jazwinski SM (1996) Longevity, genes, and aging. Science 273:54–59

Maelzer DA (1990) Fruit fly outbreaks in Adelaide, S.A., from 1948–49 to 1985–86. I. Demarcation, frequency and temporal patterns of outbreaks. Aust Zool 38:439–452

Mansingh A (1971) Physiological classification of dormancies in insects. Can Entomol 103:983–1009

Meats K, Khoo KC (1976) The dynamics of ovarian maturation and oocyte resorption in the Queensland fruit fly, *Dacus tryoni*, in daily-rhythmic and constant temperature regimes. Physiol Entomol 1:213–221

Müller H-G, Wang J-L, Capra WB, Liedo P, Carey JR (1997) Early mortality surge in protein-deprived females causes reversal of male-female life expectancy relation in Mediterranean fruit flies. Proc US Nat Acad Sci 94:2762–2765

Papadopoulos NT, Carey JR, Katsoyannos BI, Kouloussis NA (1996) Overwintering of the Mediterranean fruit fly, *Ceratitis capitata* (Diptera: Tephritidae), in Northern Greece. Ann Entomol Soc Amer 89:526–534

Partridge L (1986) Sexual activity and life span. In: Collatz KG, Sohal RS (eds) Insect aging: strategies and mechanisms. Springer-Verlag, Berlin, pp. 45–54

Partridge L, Andrews R (1985) The effect of reproductive activity on the longevity of male *Drosophila melanogaster* is not caused by an acceleration of aging. J Insect Physiol 31:393–395

Partridge L, Fowler K (1992) Direct and correlated responses to selection on age at reproduction in *Drosophila melanogaster*. Evolution 46:76–91

Pressat R (1985) The dictionary of demography. Basil Blackwell Ltd., Oxford

Ragland SS, Sohal RS (1973) Mating behavior, physical activity and aging in the housefly, *Musca domestica*. Exp Gerontol 8:135–145

Reznick D (1985) Costs of reproduction: an evaluation of the empirical evidence. Oikos 44:257–267

Rivnay E (1950) The Mediterranean fruit fly in Israel. Bull Entomol Res 41:321–341

Smith JM (1958) The effects of temperature and of egg-laying on the longevity of *Drosophila subobscura*. J Exp Biol 53:832–842

Tatar M, Carey JR, Vaupel JW (1993) Long term cost of reproduction with and without accelerated senescence in *Callosobruchus maculatus*: analysis of age-specific mortality. Evolution 47:1302–1312

Vargas RI, Harris EJ, Nishida T (1983) Distribution and seasonal occurrence of *Ceratitis capitata* (Wiedemann) (Diptera: Tephritidae) on the island of Kauai in the Hawaiian Islands. Environ Entomol 12:303–310

Vaupel JW, Carey JR, Christensen K, Johnson TE, Yashin AI, Holm NV, Iachine IA, Khazaeli AA, Liedo P, Longo VD, Yi Z, Manton KG, Curtsinger JW (1998) Biodemographic trajectories of longevity. Science, in press

Wachter K, Finch C (1997) Between Zeus and the salmon: the biodemography of longevity. National Academy Press, Washington, DC

Do the Oldest Old Grow Old More Slowly?

J. R. WILMOTH[1] and S. HORIUCHI[2]

Abstract

Although mortality rates rise exponentially through most of the adult age range in humans and many other species, it is well documented that this increase in the risk of death tends to decelerate among the oldest old. Thus, if aging is measured by the increase in mortality, it appears that the oldest old grow old more slowly. Or do they? A popular alternative hypothesis is that heterogeneity in frailty yields aggregate patterns that misrepresent age-related changes in mortality risks at the individual level. In this paper, we review arguments and evidence about the causes of mortality deceleration at older ages. We also distinguish between two fundamentally different models of heterogeneity (regarding variations in either the level or the slope of individual mortality curves), which yield opposite answers to the question posed in the title of this paper. Finally, we discuss epistemological issues affecting current explanations of mortality deceleration, including the impossibility of distinguishing conclusively between major competing hypotheses on the basis of mortality data alone.

It has commonly been observed in both human and some animal or insect populations that the risk of death tends to increase exponentially with age through some or most of the adult age range. Because of this empirical regularity, the Gompertz curve has become a standard of mortality analysis (Gompertz 1825). At some age, however, this pattern of regular exponential increase in the risk of dying tends to cease (Vaupel et al. 1998). Above this age, which may be moderately or very high depending on the species, the risk of death rises less than exponentially (that is, at a decreasing relative rate).

In studies of human mortality, this phenomenon has been referred to as "deceleration in the age pattern of mortality at older ages" (Horiuchi and Wilmoth 1998) and has been documented for a variety of populations with reliable data (Horiuchi and Coale 1990; Thatcher et al. 1998). The term "deceleration" is

[1] Department of Demography, University of California, 2232 Piedmont Avenue, Berkeley, CA 94720-2120, USA.
[2] Laboratory of Populations, Rockefeller University, 1230 York Avenue, New York, NY 10021-6399, USA.

J.-M. Robine et al. (Eds.)
Research and Perspectives in Longevity
The Paradoxes of Longevity
© Springer-Verlag Berlin Heidelberg New York 1999

especially appropriate when discussing this phenomenon in humans, since mortality rates continue to increase, though at a diminishing (relative) rate, even at the highest ages where they can be reliably measured. In insect or animal populations, more extreme forms of deceleration have occasionally been observed, including declines in death rates at very old ages (Carey et al. 1992). Some form of deceleration in the age pattern of mortality occurs in househould fruit flies (Curtsinger et al. 1992; Fukui et al. 1993), Mediterranean fruit flies (Carey et al. 1992), nematode worms (Brooks et al. 1994; Vaupel et al. 1994), bean beetles (Carey and Tatar 1994), and even American automobiles (Vaupel 1997). Furthermore, to our knowledge, no exceptions have been observed thus far: in all cases where sufficiently large populations were observed (cohorts of around 1000 individuals or more), the age-related (relative) increase in mortality decelerates at older ages.

This common finding raises fundamental questions about the nature of the aging process in humans and other species (as well as mechanical devices). Do the oldest old grow old more slowly? Based on observed mortality patterns, the answer to this question appears to be yes. Nevertheless, there are at least two points that must be considered in detail. First, what is the appropriate measure of aging for use in addressing such a question? Second, how are aggregate patterns in some measure of aging related to individual patterns? Demographers have devoted several works to the latter question but have given only scant attention to the former consideration. Here, we attempt to provide an overview of the relevant issues that must be addressed before a meaningful answer can be given to the question posed in the title of this paper.

Definitions

To avoid confusion, we begin by defining two important terms in the question we are trying to address. First, we will state what is meant by the "oldest old". Next, we will discuss the colloquial phrase employed here, "growing old," in relation to its technical counterparts, "aging" and "senescence."

Oldest Old

The term "oldest old" was coined in 1984 by Mathilda White Riley and Richard Suzman while organizing a session for the annual meeting of the American Association for the Advancement of Science (Suzman et al. 1992). It was a modification of an earlier term, the "old old," who were distinguished from the "young old" by the extent of their physical frailty and social dependence (Neugarten 1974).

In practice, it is common to define the oldest old as all persons aged 85 and over, regardless of their physical status. Although it thus loses some of its original meaning, a definition based on age is more convenient for purposes of research than one based on functional status. Furthermore, persons above age 85 are those most likely to possess characteristics that we associate with extreme old age – frailty, dependence, illness, and death (Taeuber and Rosenwaike 1992).

An alternative terminology is the "Fourth Age," which has been defined as a stage of "final dependence, decrepitude and death." In contrast, the Third Age includes individuals who are elderly but still enjoy "an era of personal fulfillment." The Third Age is a term of French origin, as in *Les Universités du Troisième Age*, which were instituted in France during the 1970s (Laslett 1991). Like the oldest old, the Fourth Age is technically a functional category, although in practice it is recognized that persons over 85 years of age are those most likely to belong to this final stage of life (Laslett 1991).

It is worth noting that most discussions employing the term "oldest old" have been with regard to human populations. The meaning and applicability of this term for non-human species are less clear.

Growing Old, Aging, and Senescence

In everyday language, "growing old" refers to the physiological deterioration that accompanies increasing age. "Aging" and "senescence" are technical terms for this same idea, although their precise definition varies from author to author. Some confusion results from the common use of "aging" in other contexts, which has led some experts to argue that it is an inappropriate term for scientific discussions (e.g., Finch 1990). For example, demographers describe the aging of populations, referring to the historical shift in the distribution of a population by age that occurs inevitably in the course of the demographic transition. Obviously, this usage is separate from the ideas we are considering here and can be put aside. In general, we should avoid using the term "aging" for physiological changes that may merely be age-related, such as the early development of an organism.

While accepting the validity of all three terms, we need to be clear about the types of internal physiological deterioration that are included in our definition of "growing old," "aging," and "senescence." An intelligent review of the varied uses of the terms "aging" and "senescence" is given by Rose (1991). For example, Rose notes that through three editions of Alex Comfort's *The Biology of Senescence*, the definition of aging did not change. According to Comfort, aging is "a progressive increase throughout life, or after a given stadium, in the likelihood that a given individual will die during the next succeeding unit of time, from randomly distributed causes ..." (cited in Rose 1991, p. 19). Thus aging, as defined by Comfort, is synonymous with the increased likelihood of death with advancing age.

Like Rose, we agree that "aging" and "senescence" (plus, we add, "growing old") refer to essentially the same concept, but we do not adopt Rose's formal definition of aging since it is based on the notion of "fitness." For Rose and other evolutionary biologists, aging or senescence includes, as a defining element, the decline of fertility as well as the increase in mortality that occurs in most older organisms. Clearly, to explain the historical development of these phenomena, it is necessary to consider the joint evolution of age patterns of death and reproduction. However, to answer the question we have posed, and to understand the mechanisms of physiological deterioration leading ultimately to death, the inclusion of reproductive decline as a privileged dimension in a general definition of aging seems inappropriate. Nevertheless, reproductive decline may be one aspect of a complex process of aging, as suggested by the finding that earlier age at natural menopause is associated with a higher age-adjusted risk of death (Snowdon et al. 1989).

Unlike Comfort, we do not limit our definition of aging to the increasing likelihood of death. Rather, in more general terms, "aging" (like "senescence" or "growing old") refers to the physiological deterioration that accompanies increasing age, raising the risk of death from a variety of causes.[3] So defined, the increase in the death rate with age is merely an indicator of aging, not its fundamental essence. In the following section, we will discuss other potential measures of aging that are consistent with this definition.

Measuring the Rate of Aging

To address questions about the age pattern of physiological deterioration in humans or other species, it is necessary to propose specific measures of the rate of aging over the life course. There are various candidates for such measures, but all involve implicit choices about the variable employed, its temporal dimension, and its level of aggregation. The life table aging rate (LAR), a convenient general-purpose measure of aging that we have used previously (Horiuchi and Coale 1990; Horiuchi and Wilmoth 1997, 1998), reflects a specific set of choices for each of these aspects, as discussed later in this section.

Choice of Variable

Most notions of aging employed in gerontology are based on the risk of death, as reflected earlier in Comfort's definition of the term. Havighurst and Sacher (1986), for example, discuss prospects for extending the length of (human) life through changes either in the "rate of aging" or in "vigor." These two concepts are defined mathematically as the slope and intercept, respectively, of a line fit to the logarithm of age-specific death rates. The authors mention two potential means of slowing the rate of aging (dietary restriction and reduced body temperature), although they are not enthusiastic about either prospect in humans. Instead, they emphasize interventions to promote increased vigor, including improvements in health services and personal habits. As they observe, increased

---

[3] This definition is close to the definition of "senescence" given by Finch (1990).

vigor would have its greatest effect on survivorship in the middle adult years (ages 40–65), whereas slowing the rate of aging would have its greatest effect on survivorship in the late adult years (after age 65).

One potential problem associated with defining the rate of aging in terms of the slope of a mortality curve is that, in some of the insect studies cited earlier, death rates are roughly constant over a significant portion of later life. A logical inference based on this measure would be that no aging occurs at these ages for these species. Whether such a conclusion is valid depends on whether there are other physiological changes occurring in individual flies during the period of constant mortality that may affect the risk of dying at some future age.

Alternatively, a measure of aging could be based on other indicators of physiological status. The presence of disease (morbidity) or functional status (disability) are two such possibilities. For flies, we might record changes with age in flight activity. In humans, several researchers have tracked the progression of specific diseases of the decline of competence in the Activities of Daily Living, or ADLs (Katz et al. 1963). Any of these age-related changes can be considered valid measures of aging by our previous definition, if there is some reason to believe that they are associated (at least eventually) with an increased risk of death for the individual.

Similarly, the rate of aging could be defined by changes in the value of various physiological parameters, often referred to as "biomarkers of aging," if such changes are thought to lead (at least eventually) to an increased risk of death. For example, it is known that bone density declines with age, especially for adult women, and that this change is associated with an increased risk of death (Ensrud et al. 1995). Therefore, physiological changes of this nature, even if they do not represent a specific morbid condition, are valid candidates for a measure of the rate of aging.

Some evolutionary biologists have proposed that "reproductive value" (i.e., the expected number of future offspring for a woman of a given age) is an appropriate measure of the rate of aging (Partridge and Barton 1993; Partridge 1997). According to the definition of aging used here, such a choice would be justifiable only to the extent that hormonal and other physiological changes associated with reproductive decline contributed to an increased probability of death (either at that moment or later in life). However, this measure of aging is also problematic in view of the fact that the "reproductive value" of a woman is zero (and thus constant) after menopause, implying a cessation of aging well before the end of the average life span.

Temporal Dimension

There are at least three aspects of the temporal dimension of measurement that deserve consideration. After choosing some parameter of physiological status to serve as a measure of aging, it is necessary to make decisions about the form in which to express age-related changes in that variable. For example, in the case of a population-based measure of disease or some chronic condition (including death), we must choose between prevalence (proportion of the population affected at some age) and incidence (rate of occurrence of new cases). Either measure can be tracked over age or time, but each offers different perspectives on the time pattern of physiological change. In general, since incidence expresses the rate of change in the prevalence of a disease or condition, the incidence rate is the more appropriate choice for a measure of aging. Furthermore, since disease occurs across the age range, it is the age-specific change (typically an increase) in the incidence rate itself that should serve as a measure of the rate of aging. In the case of mortality, this means the rate of increase with age in the death rate.

In addition, we must choose between measures of aging that are constant across the age range and ones that vary with age. As noted earlier, some authors have used the slope of a line fitted to the logarithm of age-specific death rates (over some portion of the adult age range) as a measure of the rate of aging (Havighurst and Sacher 1986). Alternatively, it is possible to estimate the slope (i.e., derivative) of this same mortality curve at each age and thus to observe changes in the rate of aging across the age range (Horiuchi and Coale 1990; Horiuchi and Wilmoth 1997).

Finally, a measure of the rate of aging can based on absolute or relative changes. The rise in human mortality rates with age decelerates only in relative terms: to our knowledge, in all cases where complete and reliable data are available, mortality rates in humans continue to rise at least linearly, even at very advanced ages, so there is no deceleration in absolute terms. When considered relative to the level of mortality at a given age, however, the rate of increase in mortality rates appears nearly constant over most of the adult age range but falls off consistently among the oldest old. Nevertheless, absolute and relative rates of changes can sometimes move in the same direction as age advances. For example, in one study bone density in adult women was shown to decline more and more rapidly with advancing age, whether measured in absolute or in percentage terms (Ensrud et al. 1995).

Level of Aggregation

Especially for the type of question asked here, it is important to distinguish between measures of aging that refer to individuals or to populations. Age-specific changes in death or incidence rates, for example, can be used to measure the rate of aging only for a population. Such measures may have a *theoretical* equivalent at the individual level (e.g., age-specific changes in the risk of death for a single person), but direct measurement of changes in underlying risks over the life of an individual is impossible. Similar limitations affect the study of age patterns of morbidity or disability in individuals. On the other hand, biomarkers of physiological status can be measured in individuals and then averaged across the population. Therefore, as argued later in this paper, measures of aging based on physiological parameters whose age-specific changes can be observed in individuals offer the only hope for comparing rates of aging at different levels of aggregation.

Life Table Aging Rate (LAR)

At the population level, a convenient and sensible measure of the rate of aging is the life table aging rate (LAR), which is defined as the relative rate of change in age-specific mortality rates with age. If μ_x is the force of mortality (or instantaneous death rate) at exact age x, the LAR, denoted by $k(x)$, is defined as follows:

$$k(x) = \frac{\mu'(x)}{\mu(x)} = \frac{d}{dx} \ln[\mu(x)]$$

In terms of the various criteria considered above, this measure of the rate of aging is characterized by its emphasis on death, by its use of the mortality rate (a particular case of an incidence rate), by its attention to the pattern of changes across the age range, by its choice to consider relative rather than absolute changes in this variable, and by its limitation to aggregate levels of analysis.

Explanations of Mortality Deceleration

There are two broad classes of explanations for why mortality deceleration occurs in humans and other animals. The first maintains that physiological changes at the level of individuals proceed more slowly in old age. Thus, the *individual-risk hypothesis* suggests that the rate of aging (by some measure) slows down in old age, leading to a deceleration in the speed of mortality increase with age. An alternative explanation builds on the observation that all populations are heterogeneous in their susceptibility to disease and death. Thus, the *heterogeneity hypothesis* suggests that selective attrition of more frail members of a population accounts for the decelerating rise in the aggregate risk of death. If true, the heterogeneity hypothesis implies that the rate of aging (by mortality or any measure) observed for a population is an underestimate of the average rate of aging in individuals.

Evidence in support of these two hypotheses comes in many forms. Here, we will attempt a brief review. Our purpose is not to resolve which hypothesis is correct or even to review all of the existing evidence, but rather to outline the key arguments in the debate and to discuss strategies for probing this issue more deeply.

Individual-Risk Hypothesis

At the core of the individual-risk hypothesis is the idea that very elderly individuals grow old more slowly than they did in earlier life. The evidence for this hypothesis in humans comes from studies of the "rate of living" and of disease progression in elderly individuals. Possible causal explanations are derived from evolutionary biology and reliability engineering. Some animal studies seem to support this hypothesis.

Rate of Living

It is well known that life spans tend to be inversely correlated across species with average metabolic rates (Finch 1990; Sohal 1986; Pearl 1928). Within species, it is sometimes observed that high levels of activity, which are associated with relatively high metabolic rates over individual lifetimes, yield shortened life spans (Sohal 1986). Therefore, it seems reasonable to examine whether the "rate of living" in elderly individuals slows down. Indeed, declines in the rate of living in old age have been observed for a number of metabolic functions (Masoro 1985), and for such fundamental processes as cell division (Grove and Kligman 1983), RNA synthesis, and protein synthesis (Remmen et al. 1995).

Disease Progression

Is has also been observed that rates of disease progression slow down at advanced ages, particularly for cancers. O'Rourke and colleagues (1987) showed that, among lung cancer patients, severity of the disease at time of diagnosis decreases with age of patient. Similarly, Peer and collaborators (1993) showed that the growth rate of primary breast cancers is significantly lower in older patients: doubling times were 80, 157, and 188 days for women under age 50, ages 50–70, and over age 70, respectively. Studies in mice confirm that some, though not all cancers, grow more slowly in elderly individuals (Kaesberg and Ershler 1989).

Evolutionary Biology

The standard prediction of evolutionary biology is that mortality rates should rise during the reproductive age range, as individuals gradually lose "reproductive value." Theoretically, since post-reproductive individuals contribute little, if anything, to the propagation of the species, there is nothing to prevent the accumulation (in evolutionary time) of deleterious mutations that serve to cull the ranks of the elderly in any species. This argument says little, however, about whether mortality rates should continue increasing rapidly at very old ages. Mueller and Rose (1996) have attempted to fill this gap in the theory based on a computer simulation of the evolution of senescence. Their simulation results yield life tables with a steep mortality increase during reproductive ages but a slowdown of mortality increase at very old ages. These findings, although addressing what seems to be a fundamental element of the evolutionary theory of life span, have been questioned by other evolutionary biologists (Charlesworth and Partridge 1997; Pletcher and Curtsinger 1998).

Reliability Engineering

In contrast to the phylogenetic perspective of evolutionary biology, reliability engineering provides an ontogenetic approach for addressing theoretical aspects of aging in humans and other species, including the phenomenon of mortality deceleration. In other words, the purpose here is not to explain *why* mortality deceleration exists, but rather to elucidate *how* it occurs. For example, Gavrilov and Gavrilova (1991) propose a simple stochastic model in which a system fails when all components of any one of its major subsystems (e. g., organs) fails. Although rates of failure for each component are constant, the failure rate for the full system rises exponentially at first and then levels off, in a manner that mimics observed patterns of mortality deceleration.

Following a different approach, Le Bras (1976) developed a simple stochastic model in which individuals move stepwise, but irreversibly, toward states that have both higher risks of failure and higher rates of further transition. Although fundamentally different in derivation, Le Bras' model implies the same pattern of failure over the life course as a simple model of heterogeneity-induced deceleration (Yashin et al. 1994).

Animal Studies

There is some rather limited evidence from animal or insect studies in support of the individual-risk hypothesis. A common strategy has been to examine the age pattern of mortality in genetically homogeneous populations of laboratory insects or worms. For example, Curtsinger et al. (1992) showed that age-specific mortality rates level off about 30 days after emergence even for genetically homogeneous cohorts of *Drosophila melanogaster* raised under favorable conditions. Such findings seem to support the individual-risk hypothesis. However, similar studies in the case of nematode worms suggest mortality deceleration at older ages is the result of population heterogeneity (Brooks et al. 1994), as discussed later.

Nevertheless, even a consistent finding of mortality deceleration among genetically homogeneous populations would not provide conclusive proof of the individual-risk hypothesis, because some sorts of heterogeneity may be acquired over the life course. Economos (1982; as cited in Curtsinger et al. 1992, p. 463) has noted "the degree of dissimilarity of individuals, even in inbred populations, all with the same age, particularly in the age-range of appreciable or high mortality. Rather small initial phenotypic differences at young age have been greatly amplified as the individuals aged." In a similar vein, Vaupel (1997, p. 25) acknowledges that in some of the various laboratory experiments measuring life spans of flies and worms, "strong efforts were made to ensure that all individuals in the population were genetically identical and that environmental conditions were highly similar for all individuals. Even in these experiments, however, individuals differed from each other, in size, in weight, and, more generally, in robustness and vitality." This result is not surprising, however, since substantial phenotypic differences are observed at birth even for genetically identical mice, suggesting that stochastic variations in prenatal development and/or environment are an important source of individual differences (Finch 1997).

Heterogeneity Hypothesis

The heterogeneity hypothesis asserts that at least some portion of the observed mortality deceleration is due to changes in the composition of a population as it grows older. The hypothesis can be illustrated using mathematical models or simulations. Some predictions of the heterogeneity hypothesis have been confirmed using aggregate mortality data. The hypothesis derives additional support from studies of the correlation of disease patterns and mortality levels within families in general, and within pairs of identical twins in particular. Both the presence of heterogeneity and the strength of its effects are suggested by studies of the age pattern of risk factors, diseases, and health status. Finally, animal studies illustrate that heterogeneity can indeed cause or accentuate mortality deceleration.

Mathematical Models

A number of mathematical studies over the past few decades have illustrated that mortality deceleration at older ages may be the result of selective attrition in a heterogeneous population (Beard 1959, 1961; Vaupel et al. 1979; Manton et al. 1986; Horiuchi and Coale 1990; Yashin et al. 1994). It is now well known that the logistic mortality curve first proposed by Perks (1932) can be derived by assuming that the force of mortality for individuals follows the Makeham (1867) curve scaled by a "frailty" parameter that follows the gamma distribution. Thus, for an individual with frailty z, the risk of death at exact age x is

$$\mu(x, z) = A + z \cdot Be^{\theta x},$$

where A, B, and θ are the standard parameters of the Makeham model, and where z represents the relative frailty of an individual and follows a gamma distribution in the population. This model is now referred to as the gamma-Makeham mortality model, and it implies that mortality at older ages approaches a constant level (i.e., a logistic model). Yashin et al. (1994) showed mathematically that two models of heterogeneity (fixed genetic differences, or variable acquired differences) yield the same age pattern of mortality.

Simulation Studies

Strehler and Mildvan (1960) and Redington (1969) simulated age patterns of cohort mortality assuming that a cohort contains subgroups whose mortality follows the Gompertz curve but with different parameter values. Notable mortality decelerations were observed in the simulated age-specific death rates for the population, which deviated considerably from the underlying Gompertz pattern. Likewise, Vaupel and Carey (1993) used simulation to reproduce the mortality deceleration observed in a large cohort of Mediterranean fruit flies. In this case, however, the authors argued that the magnitude of heterogeneity required to yield the observed pattern was implausibly large, and thus that heterogeneity could not be the sole explanation of the mortality deceleration observed.

Empirical Predictions

It is possible to test certain predictions of the heterogeneity hypothesis using aggregate mortality data. Specifically, as we have argued previously, the heterogeneity hypothesis implies: 1) decelerations for most major causes of death, 2) decelerations starting at younger ages for more "selective" causes, and 3) a shift of the deceleration to older ages with declining levels of mortality. In a detailed analysis of mortality data for Sweden, 1861–1990, and Japan, 1951–1990, these three predictions were largely confirmed (Horiuchi and Wilmoth 1998). However, these predictions may also be consistent with various versions of the individual-risk hypothesis, which is quite flexible and compatible with almost any observed pattern. Nevertheless, if our empirical study had been inconsistent with these three predictions, the heterogeneity hypothesis would have been rejected. Having passed these tests, it gains some credibility.

As further confirmation, our ongoing work shows that the deceleration pattern has shifted to older ages (by about 10 years of age) during the last few decades for women in many industrialized countries. (This shift is less clear in males, whose mortality declines have been less pronounced and whose age patterns of mortality are confounded with strong cohort variations due to cumulative effects of smoking and long-term health impacts of the World Wars.) An explanation of this phenomenon in terms of individual risk is that the senescence schedule has shifted by 10 years: for example, the contention that 80-year-old women today are aging like their 70-year-old counterparts a few decades ago. Although there is some evidence of recent health improvements among the elderly (Manton et al. 1997; Crimmins et al. 1997), this interpretation needs additional support, since there is other evidence that the timing of the aging process in women has not changed significantly: for example, the fact that the average age at menopause has been nearly constant during this period. Therefore, at the present time, the most plausible explanation for the phenomenon of a shift in mortality deceleration to older ages is given by the heterogeneity hypothesis.

Twin and Family Studies

Genetic variation is surely one cause of heterogeneity in the risk of death in a population, but how large are these differences? In general, we know from statistical models employed in twin studies that roughly one quarter of the intra-population variability in individual ages at death may be due to genetic factors (McGue et al. 1993; Herskind et al. 1996). Furthermore, the genetic basis of specific risks due to coronary heart disease (CHD) has been amply demonstrated by a series of studies involving twins or family members. For example, Marenberg and colleagues (1994), in a study of Swedish twins, showed that the relative risk of death from CHD increases substantially for individuals whose twin died of CHD at a relatively young age. Other studies also document the elevated risk of CHD for persons with a family history of the aliment (Colditz et al. 1986; Schild-kraut et al. 1989).

Risk Factors and Diseases

The genetic component of heart disease is related in part to differences in major risk factors, like cholesterol. For example, a study of Swedish twins reared apart showed that an individual's total cholesterol level is heavily influenced by genetic mechanisms (Heller et al. 1993). A related finding is that specific genes influence the risk of heart attack and the subsequent probability of survival. For example, Kramer and colleagues (1991) showed a sharp drop with age in the prevalence of the deficient, silent allotype of the C4B gene (C4B*Q0), suggesting that it is a probable negative selection factor for survival. In a later study, they also showed an association between myocardial infarction and the presence of this same allotype, especially in men (Kramer et al. 1994). Not only was C4B*Q0 significantly more common in men presenting with myocardial infarction than in healthy controls, but also carrier state was shown to influence the outcome of a myocardial infarction (percent surviving was 50, 79, or 80, for homozygous, heterozygous, or non-carriers, respectively).

Similarly, recent work documents an important genetic component in rates of disease and death due to Alzheimer's dementia (AD). Corder and colleagues (1993) showed an association between AD and the presence of the APOE-ε4 allele on chromosome 19. Although the APOE-ε4 allele has a much larger effect on AD morbidity than mortality, its selective effect is still evident. Furthermore, several studies have shown that the prevalence of the APOE-ε4 allele decreases with age among individuals with or without AD (Rebeck et al. 1994; Loujiha et al. 1994).

Health Status of Oldest Old

It has often been observed that survivors to extreme old age are sometimes healthier, both mentally and physically, than those who died at younger ages. This observation seems to support the idea that mortality deceleration occurs because of the selective action of mortality itself. For example, one study showed that men in their 90s have higher levels of cognitive function, on average, than men in their 80s (Perls et al. 1993). The anomaly is due to selective mortality, since the risk of death among older men varies considerably in relation to cognitive performance. A similar result was not found for women, perhaps because selective survival is more pronounced for men than for women of the same age due to higher death rates.

Animal Studies

As noted earlier, experimental studies involving household fruit flies suggest that genetic heterogeneity is sometimes inadequate as an explanation of mortality deceleration, since the phenomenon is observed in genetically homogeneous populations as well. On the other hand, mortality rates for isogenic strains of nematode worms (*Caenorhabditis elegans*) show an exponential pattern of increase that does not decelerate in later life (Brooks et al. 1994). In genetically heterogeneous populations, however, death rates for these worms increase exponentially through the first 17 days of life, but then level off and remain almost constant until the last death occurs at about 60 days.[4] These results suggest that late-life mortality deceleration in nematode worms may be mostly a function of genetic heterogeneity in the risk of death.

Two Types of Heterogeneity

As reviewed in the previous section, one explanation for observed patterns of mortality deceleration is a change in the composition of the population with age. In this section, we explore two versions of the heterogeneity hypothesis and discuss their implications.

---

[4] Vaupel et al. (1994), reanalyzing the data of Brooks et al. (1994), document a deceleration in the age pattern of mortality for *C. elegans* fairly early in life (around day 8, when survival proportions still exceed 90 percent), even in genetically homogeneous populations of worms. However, this finding does not contradict the key result of Brooks and colleagues, who showed that mortality deceleration *during later life* (after day 17) in a genetically heterogeneous population of nematode worms is indeed due to selective attrition.

Slope versus Level

In the most common version of the heterogeneity hypothesis, survivors to old age grow old at the same rate as their peers, but their risk of death is simply lower, on average, throughout life. We refer to this model as "level hertogeneity," since it implies differences among individuals in the level of mortality risks throughout life but no differences in the rate of aging. Mortality risks that differ by level only can be represented by the following equation:

$$\mu(x, z) = z \cdot \mu_0(x),$$

where $\mu_0(x)$ is the baseline hazard function and z is the relative frailty for a given individual. This is the well-known proportional hazards model in its simplest form. If the baseline hazard is represented by the Gompertz curve, the model becomes:

$$\mu(x, z) = z \cdot Be^{\theta x}.$$

It is also possible, however, that individuals differ in their rate of mortality increase with age, suggesting a model that we refer to as "slope heterogeneity." Suppose, for example, that mortality risks due to aging are equivalent in a popu-

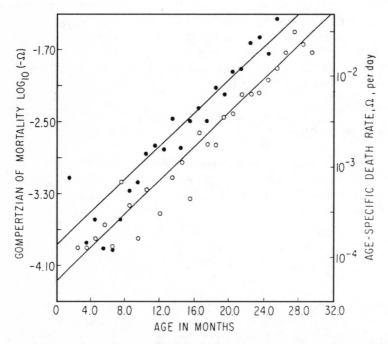

Fig. 1. Gompertz curves for control (solid circles) and procaine-treated rats (open circles). Parallelism shows that procaine prolongs life span by reducing vulnerability across the age range without changing the rate of aging. Original graph is from Sacher (1977); also reproduced in Arking (1991)

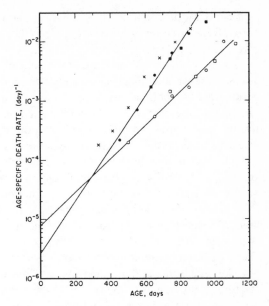

Fig. 2. Gompertz curves for control (closed symbols and crosses) and rats subject to caloric restriction (open symbols). Different slopes show that dietary restriction prolongs life span by reducing the rate of aging. Original graph is from Sacher (1977); also reproduced in Arking (1991).

lation at the time of sexual maturity (around 12–13 years in humans) but that their rate of increase with age differs among individuals. In the case of Gompertz mortality, such a model is represented by the following equation:

$$\mu(x, z) = Be^{z \cdot \theta(x-12.5)}.$$

There is some experimental support for the plausibility of such a model. For example, differences in slope have been observed among groups of nematode worms (Johnson 1990), fruit flies (Orr and Sohal 1994), and mice (Sacher 1956). In all cases, the individuals either differ genetically or are exposed to different experimental conditions.

Figures 1 and 2 provide examples of experimental data that are consistent with each of these two models (originally from Sacher 1977, who provides references for the data; the same comparison appears in Arking 1991). In laboratory rats, two experimental manipulations were shown to prolong life span, but the timing of their effects was fundamentally different. In one case, rats treated with procaine enjoy a reduced risk of dying that is of similar magnitude across the life course. In the other example, rats subjected to caloric restriction show a progressively larger mortality advantage with advancing age – thus, they appear to age more slowly.

Interpretation

It is easy to confirm via simulation that each of the two heterogeneity models (or combinations of them) provides a possible explanation for the phenomenon of mortality deceleration in humans (Horiuchi and Wilmoth 1998). Each suggests that deceleration is due to changes in the composition of the elderly population through the attrition of mortality itself, rather than to a slowdown in the rate of physiological deterioration (aging) at older ages. However, the two types of heterogeneity yield opposite answers to the question posed in the title of this paper. In the case of level heterogeneity, all individuals grow old at the same rate throughout life, and mortality deceleration is merely the result of compositional changes. In the case of slope heterogeneity, on the other hand, survivors to old age do indeed grow old more slowly than their peers who have died, because the selective attrition of mortality removes individuals who are aging more rapidly.

The distinction between "level" and "slope" heterogeneity is important, though we have not yet fully explored its implications. At least one previous study has argued, for example, that the amount of heterogeneity required to produce some observed empirical patterns is implausibly large (Vaupel and Carey 1993). However, this study and almost all others that employ formal models of heterogeneity in the risk of death have examined variations in the level, but not the slope, on individual mortality trajectories.

Common sense and our own anecdotal observations suggest that heterogeneity among individuals in the rate of aging is at least as plausible as constant (proportional) differences in mortality risks. Furthermore, since differences in the slope of individual mortality curves are associated with an increasing disparity between individual mortality risks with age, it is possible that explanations of empirical findings that seem implausible under a hypothesis of level heterogeneity might appear more plausible under an assumption of slope heterogeneity.

Testing the Individual-Risk Hypothesis

Most studies of mortality deceleration in humans have focused on the heterogeneity hypothesis. The strategy has been to determine whether observed patterns could plausibly be explained by heterogeneity among individuals in the risk of death. In general, at least for humans, heterogeneity appears to offer a quite plausible explanation for mortality deceleration (Horiuchi and Wilmoth 1998). The problem with this line of work is that the merits of the major alternative explanation, the individual-risk hypothesis, are not fully explored.

For example, the premise of our recent extensive analysis of Swedish and Japanese historical mortality patterns was that the heterogeneity hypothesis carries certain logical implications, or predictions. Our strategy was to determine whether these predictions are confirmed by empirical observations. These predictions were not trivial, and there was no reason to believe *a priori* that they would be fulfilled. For the most part, the specific predictions of the heterogeneity hypothesis that we put forward were confirmed by empirical analysis. However, although these findings bolster the heterogeneity hypothesis as a plausible explanation of mortality deceleration, they do not allow us to reject the alternative explanation offered by the individual-risk hypothesis. In fact, the individual-risk hypothesis is quite flexible and consistent with almost any conceivable mortality pattern. Thus, it is difficult, if not impossible, to propose falsifiable tests of the individual-risk hypothesis based on mortality data alone.

Therefore, in this section, we discuss strategies for testing the individual-risk hypothesis. We do not claim to have resolved these issues or pretend that these strategies will be easy to implement. Rather, we are attempting merely to define the necessary conditions for testing the individual-risk hypothesis.

Choice of Variables

The first requirement for testing the individual-risk hypothesis is to choose variables that provide comparable measures of aging at both individual and aggregate levels. For this purpose, data on mortality alone are clearly inadequate. Models of population heterogeneity, as discussed earlier, assume implicitly that each person in the population possesses an individual mortality curve, $\mu(x, z)$, which is a function of both age, x, and relative frailty, z. Thus, the time at death for each individual is a random variable with its own probability distribution. This assumption is not unreasonable on its own. One difficulty posed by this model, however, is that it is impossible to estimate the underlying mortality curve for an individual based on information about a single time at death. Since there are no direct estimates of individual mortality curves (only an assumption that these curves are proportional to one another), we have no means of testing the individual-risk hypothesis using mortality data alone.

Of course, it is possible to estimate the *average* lifetime risk of death for an individual given the time at death. In this case, a maximum likelihood estimate of the average risk is merely the reciprocal of the survival time. Nevertheless, this model is different from the one stated earlier, since it assumes a constant lifetime mortality risk and thus no aging. It seems that the only means of measuring directly the *age pattern* of individual mortality risks is to analyze death times for large populations of genetically identical persons, or clones. From studies of inbred lines of insects and worms, however, we know that heterogeneity may persist even in these populations in the form of acquired differences.

We reject, therefore, the notion that the individual-risk hypothesis could be either accepted or rejected based on mortality data alone. To test this hypothesis properly, it will be necessary to choose variables, and hence measures of aging, other than mortality. Unfortunately, most common measures of morbidity and disability suffer from similar deficiencies, since they too are defined by dichotomous (or polytomous) categories that do not generally yield continuous measures of the progression of aging in individuals.

Theoretically, if the progression through states of disease and disability were defined and measured in great detail, they would more closely approximate the underlying physiological changes associated with aging. Thus, some very detailed measures of morbidity or functionality might prove to be legitimate sources of information on the rate of aging in individuals. Current notions of disease and disability, however, are too specific for this purpose, capturing only the final stages of physiological deterioration, and thus do not provide a viable means of defining or measuring aging over the life course of individuals.

If aging in individuals cannot be measured by mortality, morbidity, or disability, then how can it be measured? The final class of measures considered here, called "biomarkers of aging" or simply "biomarkers," seems to offer the best hope for this purpose. By definition, biomarkers are measures of an individual's physiological characteristics that can be measured continuously over the life course. Therefore, it is possible to compare changes in physiological status for individuals to the average changes for a population.

Familiar examples of biomarkers in humans include blood glucose, serum cholesterol, vital capacity index, body mass index, hematocrit, diastolic and systolic blood pressure, cardiac function, and ventricular rate (Manton et al. 1994). Age variations in various biomarkers have been investigated in a number of gerontological and geriatric studies (e.g., Balin 1994; Masoro 1995; Shock et al. 1984; Timiras 1994). All such indicators of physiological status are measurable continuously over the life of individuals, and their typical age-related changes are known to be associated with increasing risks of morbidity and mortality. Therefore, these variables can provide a rich source of information about the rate of aging. Furthermore, because they are directly measurable in individuals, they permit a comparison of individual and aggregate patterns of aging.

Nevertheless, some caution is in order regarding the promises and pitfalls of biomarker research. The goal of finding reliable measures of physiological aging in individuals is not universally viewed as feasible or even desirable. Masoro (1988) claims that the controversy revolves around two major issues: first, a lack of knowledge about basic aging processes, and second, a lack of clarity about what a biomarker of aging is designed to do. Let us consider each of these issues.

A key point of controversy in biomarker research is the general scientific uncertainty about whether aging is a unitary or a multidimensional process. Thus, it is unknown whether all aging processes proceed at the same rate within a single individual, linked somehow to a single causal mechanism, or whether individuals age more or less slowly depending on the characteristic being considered.[5] Rather than abandoning the enterprise because of this difficulty, it seems that careful studies of biomarkers of aging should be viewed as one means of resolving this central question in aging research. The task will not be easy, however, especially given the degree of noise in the variables being measured. Miller (1997) notes, for example, that T cell subsets, though "robustly age-sensitive," are also influenced by genetic polymorphisms, chronic and acute stresses, irradiation, medication, and infectious agents. Therefore, one can only hope that beneath the layers of noise it will be possible to uncover the nature of the statistical associations among different biomarkers of aging. Even if not perfectly correlated

---

[5] The age pattern of mortality differs significantly among major degenerative diseases (Horiuchi and Wilmoth 1997). A possible reason for this diversity is that aging processes underlying those diseases may not be highly orchestrated.

(which is impossible, in any case, due to noise), their pattern of variation might be described using a small number of dimensions.

But what constitutes a valid biomarker of aging? Miller (1997, p. 1262) sets a high standard: "Merely showing that a given assay changes with age, and thus distinguishes most old people from most young people is not sufficient to qualify a test as a biomarker. What counts is showing that the test in question divides people (or mice) of a given age into groups that differ predictably in a wide range of other age-sensitive traits." In other words, biomarkers of aging should differentiate the young from the old, but they should also be correlated, such that individuals of a given age who are "old" with respect to one trait tend to be "old" with respect to other traits as well. While this is an admirable goal, the required correlation seems to assume the existence of a single underlying aging process and may need to be reviewed as further evidence emerges about the dimensionality of aging. It may be, for example, that some valid biomarkers of aging are correlated at some ages but not at others, either because of an underlying multi-dimensionality or because of age patterns in the noise.

Regardless of the precise definition, it is important to remember that not all risk factors qualify as valid biomarkers of aging. For example, smoking increases one's risk of mortality, but smoking status does not change predictably as a function of age, and it may or may not be correlated (at a given age) with measures of aging. Miller (1997, p. 1262) argues: "Showing that an assay not only predicts subsequent mortality but also correlates in plausible ways with other age-sensitive traits is a minimal standard to which proposed biomarkers must be held." Thus, ideally, biomarkers of aging should 1) predict subsequent mortality and 2) be correlated at a given age in a manner that is consistent with their age-related changes. As noted already, however, the second requirement may have to be modified as our knowledge of fundamental processes improves.

Concerning the goals of biomarker research, we propose that a central purpose should be to measure the rate of aging in individuals and thus to describe differences in the rate of aging within population, across species, and over the life course. Although formal documentation of the rate of aging in individuals will not resolve all the mysteries of aging, such results should provide clues about how to proceed in other areas of aging research. Measuring the rate of aging is only one possible goal of biomarker research, and there may be other worthwhile goals as well. An earlier application used biomarkers of aging as a means of calculating the "functional" or "biological" age of individuals (as distinct from their chronological age), but this concept has been strongly criticized, and perhaps for good reason (Costa and McCrae 1985). Time will tell whether other applications of biomarker research suffer a similar fate. Nevertheless, we should find cause for optimism in recent advances in biomarker research involving mice and monkeys (Miller et al. 1997; Short et al. 1997).

Models of Mortality and Physiological Decline

Of course, the relationship between various biomarkers of aging and ultimate outcomes, such as morbidity and mortality, is not fully understood. Thus, it would be imprudent to adopt a general definition of aging based on a certain set of variables merely because those variables can be conveniently measured in individuals. It is also important to recall the strong intuitive appeal of defining aging in terms of the age pattern of mortality, which is, after all, a singularly important event in the lifetime of any individual. In spite of the difficulties in defining the concept, it is generally acknowledged that aging is a complex process with, nonetheless, only one ultimate outcome, death.

Thus, the challenge to scientists working in this area is to specify models that retain the traditional definition of the rate of aging in terms of increasing mortality risks, but that still permit a comparison of rates of aging at the individual and aggregate levels by incorporating measures of physiological status in individuals. Some previous research has been done on modeling the relationship between biomarkers and mortality, including the pioneering work of Strehler and Mildvan (1960), Sacher and Trucco (1962), and Brown and Forbes (1974 a, b, 1975, 1976), as well as the more recent work of Manton and colleagues (1994). In these modeling exercises, however, it is important to maintain clarity about the goals of the research. The practice of treating biomarkers of aging and risk factors (e.g., smoking) in an equivalent manner is questionable. Likewise, proportional hazards models (even in the presence of time-varying covariates) provide a rather limited analytical framework if our purpose is to understand the rate of aging.

Of course, all models that would permit a comparison of individual and aggregate trajectories of age-related variables must include some provision for heterogeneity. As discussed before, this heterogeneity can take on more than one form. Additional data on various indicators of physiological change in individuals should provide some basis for deciding how to incorporate heterogeneity into these models. It should be possible, for example, to distinguish between slope and level heterogeneity using data on biomarkers of aging. As our empirical knowledge improves, the specifications of our mathematical models should be adjusted accordingly.

Data Sources

Obviously, a considerable difficulty in the research strategy we are proposing is that appropriate data are not generally available. Certainly, data on age trajectories have been collected for a variety of biomarkers in humans (e.g., Balin 1994; Masoro 1995; Shock et al. 1984; Timiras 1994). Most of these data, however, are not very useful for examining possible decelerations of aging processes among the oldest old for two reasons. First, they are usually obtained from cross-sectional study designs, or are derived using some mixed strategies of cross-sectional and longitudinal analyses,[6] and thus age patterns derived from them are often contaminated by selective survival. Second, the size of the elderly population included in the study is usually not large enough to permit an accurate calculation of possible differences in the rate of aging between the young old and the oldest old.

For these reasons, the number of longitudinal studies with potentially appropriate data is extremely limited. The most promising candidate is surely the Baltimore Longitudinal Study of Aging (BLSA), although the number of participants remaining at very old ages is still rather small, diminishing the amount of information available on trajectories of age-related variables over the entire adult age range.[7] Thus, whether it will be possible to answer, even in a preliminary manner, the question posed here using existing data is very much an open question.

We are inspired to move forward with this approach nevertheless, because we believe that much richer sources of data will become more widely available in the future. At least some of the information needed for analyses of the type we are proposing is contained already in the medical records of countless individuals. The difficulty, of course, is that these medical records are generally not available to researchers due to concerns about confidentiality. As such records become increasingly computerized, however, the potential for mining this rich source of information will grow. Researchers, we believe, should position themselves to be able to take advantage of this emerging situation, in a manner that safeguards the confidentiality of individual medical records while at the same time exploiting them as a valuable source of scientific data.

In addition, laboratory animals are important for testing the individual-risk hypothesis of mortality deceleration. Because of their relatively brief lives, age trajectories of their biomarkers for the entire life span can be obtained within a few weeks or years, depending on the species. Fortunately, the genetics and demography of nematodes and flies have become increasingly familiar, but there seems to have been less work in the area of physiological and biochemical measurement of individuals over the life course. Some recent work holds promise, including a technique to allow the direct observation of stress response in *C. elegans*. Since there is some evidence that changes with age in stress response are part of the normal aging process, perhaps related to oxidative damage, the technique might eventually be used to develop one or more biomarkers of aging in nematodes (Chris Link and Tom Johnson, personal communication, 1998).

Biomarker research on rodents and monkeys is more developed (Miller et al. 1997; Short et al. 1997), but to our knowledge, such data have not been collected or analyzed for the specific purpose of testing hypotheses about the age pattern of mortality. Measurement of age trajectories of biomarkers in laboratory ani-

---

[6] If the initial ages of respondents in a longitudinal study cover a wide range, age-related changes can be followed for multiple, overlapping age intervals (Elahi et al. 1996). This design is better than the regular cross-sectional design, but it is not free of selection biases nonetheless.

[7] Other important data sets include the Framingham study and the National Long Term Care Survey (NLTCS). As sources of information about biomarkers, however, these studies are more limited than the BLSA. The Framingham study focuses on indicators that are closely related to cardiovascular diseases, and the NLTCS concentrates on indicators of functional status.

mals will be considerably more costly than measurement of their mortality patterns, but this approach seems promising as a means of understanding the relationships that link different dimensions of the aging process, and that link aging to the risks of mortality and morbidity (Heller et al. 1998).

Conclusion

This paper began with a seemingly simple question: Do the oldest old grow old more slowly? It is well documented that the exponential rise in mortality rates tends to decelerate for humans and some other species at advanced ages, but does this mean that the process of aging occurs more slowly in the oldest old? If measured by the rise in aggregate death rates, the answer to these questions appears to be yes. However, aging can be measured by a variety of indicators, including but not limited to mortality rates. Furthermore, it is well known that population heterogeneity can distort aggregate age patterns relative to their individual-level counterparts.

We have reviewed arguments and evidence about the causes of mortality deceleration at older ages. We have also distinguished between two fundamentally different models of heterogeneity (regarding variations in either the level or the slope of individual mortality curves), which yield opposite answers to the question posed in our title. If individual mortality curves differ only by level (i. e., proportional hazards), then mortality deceleration may be purely an artifact of selective attrition. On the other hand, if the rate of aging is variable across the population, then survivors to advanced ages will enjoy lower rates of aging on average. In this case, the oldest old are a select group of individuals for whom aging occurs more slowly – not only in old age, but throughout their lives.

A third possible explanation for mortality deceleration is the individual-risk hypothesis, which presumes that the rate of aging for individuals slows down at advanced ages. We argue that this hypothesis cannot be adequately tested using mortality data alone and will require other sources of information, in particular, longitudinal data on biomarkers of aging. Although such data are not widely available in a convenient form at the present time, we suggest that demographers and others should develop the theoretical machinery for such analyses nevertheless, since appropriate data may become more widely available in the future.

Acknowledgments:

This paper was presented in a departmental seminar in Berkeley and at a conference in Paris sponsored by the IPSEN Foundation. The authors thank the attendees on both occasions for their helpful and encouraging comments. This research was sponsored by the National Institute on Aging (R01-AG11552, K01-AG00554, and R01-AG10518). Please send comments by email to jrw@demog.berkeley.edu.

References

Arking R (1991) Biology of aging: observations and principles. Engelwood Cliffs, Prentice Hall

Balin AK (ed) (1994) Practical handbook of human biologic age determination. Boca Raton, CRC Press

Beard RE (1959) Note on some mathematical mortality models. CIBA Foundation colloquia on ageing. Vol. 5. The life span of animals. Wolstenholme GEW, O'Connor M (eds) Boston, Little, Brown and Company, 302–311

Beard RE (1961) A theory of mortality based on actuarial, biological and medical considerations. International Population Conference, New York. London, IUSSP

Brooks A, Lithgow GJ, Johnson TE (1994) Mortality rates in a genetically heterogeneous population of *Caenorhabditis elegans*. Science 263:668–671

Brown KS, Forbes WF (1974 a) A mathematical model of aging process. J. Gerontol 29:46–51

Brown KS, Forbes WF (1974 b) A mathematical model of aging process II. J. Gerontol 29:401–409

Brown KS, Forbes WF (1975) A mathematical model of aging process III. J. Gerontol 30:513–525

Brown KS, Forbes WF (1976) A mathematical model of aging process IV. K- Gerontol 31:385–395

Carey JR, Tatar M (1994) Sex mortality differentials in the bean beetle: reframing the question. Am Natural 144:165–175

Carey JR, Liedo P, Orozco D, Vaupel JW (1992) Slowing of mortality rates at older ages in large medfly cohorts. Science 258:457–463

Charlesworth B, Partridge L (1997) Ageing: levelling of the grim reaper. Curr Biol 7:R440–R442

Colditz GA, Stampfer MJ, Willett WC, Rosner B, Speizer FE, Hennekens CH (1986) A prospective study of parental history of myocardial infarction and coronary heart disease in women. Am J Epidemiol 123:48–58

Comfort A (1969) Test-battery to measure ageing-rate in man. Lancet 2:1411–1415

Corder EH, Saunders AM, Strittmatter WJ, Schmeckel DE, Gaskell PC, Small GW, Roses AD, Haines JL, Perikal-Vance MA (1993) Apolipoprotein ε4 gene dose and the risk of Alzheimer disease in late-onset families. Science 261:921–923

Costa PT Jr, McCrae RR (1985) Concepts of functional or biological age: a critical review. Principles of geriatric medicine. Andres R, Bierman EL, Hazzard WR (eds) New York, McGraw-Hill, 30–37

Crimmins EM, Saito Y, Ingegneri D (1997) Trends in disability-free life expectancy in the U.S. Pop Develop Rev 23(3):555–572

Curtsinger JW, Fukui HH, Townsend D, Vaupel JW (1992) Demography of genotypes: failure of the limited lifespan paradigm in *Drosophila melanogaster*. Science 258:461–463

Economos AC (1982) Rate of aging, rate of dying and the mechanism of mortality. Arch Gerontol Geriat 1:3–27

Elahi D, Muller DC, Rowe JW (1996) Design, conduct, and analysis of human aging research. Handbook of the biology of aging. Fourth Edition. Schneider EL, Rowe JW (eds) New York, Academic Press, 24–36

Ensrud KE, Palermo L, Black DM, Cauley J, Jergas M, Orwoll ES, Nevitt MC, Fox KM, Cummings SR (1995) Hip and calcaneal bone loss increase with advancing age: longitudinal results from the study of osteoporotic fractures. J Bone Mineral Res 10(11):1778–1787

Finch CE (1990) Longevity, senescence and the genome. Chicago, The University of Chicago Press

Finch CE (1997) Longevity: Is everything under genetic control? An inquiry into non-genetic and non-environmental sources of variation. Longevity: to the limits and beyond. Robine J-M, Vaupel JW, Jeune B, Allard M (eds) Heidelberg, Springer-Verlag, 165–178

Fukui HH, Xiu HL, Curtsinger JW (1993) Slowing of age-specific mortality rates in *Drosophila melanogaster*. Exp Gerontol 38:585–599

Gavrilov LA, Gavrilova NS (1991) The biology of life span: a quantitative approach. New York, Harwood

Gompertz B (1825) On the nature of the function expressive of the law of human mortality. Philosophical Transactions 27:513–585

Grove GL, Kligman AM (1983) Age-associated changes in human epidermal cell renewal. J Gerontol 38:137–142

Havighurst RJ, Sacher GA (1986) Prospects of lengthening life and vigor. Extending the human life span: social policy and social ethics. Neugarten B, Havighurst R (eds) Chicago, University of Chicago Press, 13–18

Heller DA, de Faire U, Pedersen NL, Dahlén G, McClearn GE (1993) Genetic and environmental influences on serum lipid level in twins. New Engl J Med 328:1150–1156

Heller DA, Ahern FM, Stout JT, McClearn GE (1998) Mortality and biomarkers of aging in heterogeneous stock (HS) mice. J Gerontol Biol Sci 53A:B217–B230

Herskind AM, McGue M, Holm NW, Sorensen TI, Harvard B, Vaupel JW (1996) The heritability of human longevity: a population-based study of 2872 Danish twin pairs born 1870–1900. Human Genet 97:319–323

Horiuchi S, Coale AJ (1990) Age patterns of mortality for older women: an analysis using the age-specific rate of mortality change with age. Math Pop Stud 2:245–267

Horiuchi S, Wilmoth JR (1997) Age patterns of the life-table aging rate for major causes of death in Japan, 1951–1990. J Gerontol Biol Sci 52A:B67–B77

Horiuchi S, Wilmoth JR (1998) Deceleration in the age pattern of mortality at older ages. Demography 35, in press

Johnson TE (1990) Increased life-span of age-1 mutants in *Caenorhabditis elegans* and lower Gompertz rate of aging. Science 249:908–912

Kaesberg PR, Ershler WB (1989) The change in tumor aggressiveness with age: lessons from experimental animals. Sem Oncol 16:28–33

Katz S, Ford AB, Moskowitz RW, Jackson BA, Jaffe MW (1963) The index of ADL: a standardized measure of biological and psychosocial function. JAMA 185(12):914–919

Kramer J, Fulop T, Rajczy K, Anh-Tuan N, Fust G (1991) A marked drop in the incidence of the null allele of the B-gene of the 4th component of complement (C4B*Q0) in elderly subjects – C4B*Q0 as a probable negative selection factor for survival. Human Genet 86(6):595–598

Kramer J, Rajczy K, Hegyi L, Fulop T, Mohacsi A, Mezei Z, Keltai M, Blasko G, Ferenczy E, Anh-Tuan N, Fust G (1994) C4B*Q0 allotype as risk factor for myocardial infarction. Br Med J 309:313–314

Laslett P (1991) A Fresh Map of Life: The Emergence of the Third Age. Cambridge, Massachusetts, Harvard University Press.

Le Bras, H (1976) Lois de mortalité et âge limite. Population 31(3):655–691

Loujiha JH, Miettinen E, Kontula K, Tikkanen MJ, Miettinen TA, Tilvis RS (1994) Aging and genetic variation of plasma apolipoproteins: relative loss of the apolipoprotein E4 phenotype in centenarians. Arteriosclerosis Thrombosis 14:1084–1089

Makeham WM (1867) On the law of mortality. J Inst Actuaries 13:335–340, 348

Manton KG, Stallard E, Vaupel JW (1986) Alternative models for the heterogeneity of mortality risks among the aged. J. Am Stat Assoc 81:635–644

Manton KG, Stallard E, Woodbury MA, Dowd JE (1994) Time-varying covariates in models of human mortality and aging: multidimensional generalization of the Gompertz. J Gerontol 49:B169–B190

Manton KG, Corder LS, Stallard E (1997) Chronic disability trends in elderly United States populations: 1982–1994. Proc Nat Acad Sci 94:2593–2598

Marenberg ME, Risch N, Berkman LF, Floderus B, de Faire U (1994) Genetic susceptibility to death from coronary heart disease in a study of twins. New Engl J. Med 330(15):1041–1046

Masoro EJ (1985) Metabolism. Handbook of the biology of aging. Finch CE, Schneider EL (eds) New York, Van Nostrand Reinhold, 540–563

Masoro EJ (1988) Physiological system markers of aging. Exp Gerontol 23:391–394

Masoro EJ (ed) (1995) Aging. Handbook of physiology. New York, Oxford University Press: Section 11

McGue M, Vaupel JW, Holm N, Harvard B (1993) Longevity is moderately heritable in a sample of Danish twins born 1870–80. J Gerontol 48:B237–B244

Miller RA (1997) When will the biology of aging become useful? Future landmarks in biomedical gerontology. J Am Geriat Soc 45:1258–1267

Miller RA, Chrisp C, Galecki A (1997) CD4 memory T cell levels predict life span in genetically heterogeneous mice. FASEB J 11:775–783

Mueller LD, Rose MR (1996) Evolutionary theory predicts late-life mortality plateaus. Proc Nat Acad Sci 93:15249–15253

Neugarten BL (1974) Age groups in American society. Daedalus 115(1):31–49

O'Rourke MA, Feussner JR, Feigl P, Laszlo J (1987) Age trends of lung cancer stage at diagnosis. JAMA 258:921–926

Orr WC, Sohal RS (1994) Extension of life-span by overexpression of superoxide dismutase and catalase in *Drosophila melanogaster*. Science 263(5150):1128–1130

Partridge L, Barton NH (1993) Evolution of aging: testing the theory using *Drosophila*. Genetica 91:89–98

Partridge L (1997) Evolutionary biology and age-related mortality. Between Zeus and the Salmon: The Biodemography of Longevity. Wachter KW, Finch CE (eds) Washington, DC, National Academy Press, 78–95

Pearl RA (1928) The rate of living. New York, Knopf

Peer PGM, van Dijck JAAM, Hendriks JHCL, Holland R, Verbeek ALM (1993) Age-dependent growth rate of primary breast cancer. Cancer 71:3547–3551

Perks W (1932) On some experiments in the graduation of mortality statistics. J Inst Actuaries 63:12–40

Perls TT, Morris JN, Ooi WL, Lipsitz LA (1993) The relationship between age, gender and cognitive performance in the very old: the effect of selective survival. J Am Geriat Soc 41:1193–1201

Pletcher SD, Curtsinger JW (1998) Mortality plateaus and the evolution of senescence: why are old-age mortality rates so low? Evolution 52:454–464

Rebeck GW, Perls TT, West HL, Sodhi P, Lipsitz LA, Hyman BT (1994) Reduced apolipoprotein ε4 allele frequency in the oldest old Alzheimer's patients and cognitively normal individuals. Neurology 44(8):1513–1516

Redington FM (1969) An exploration into patterns of mortality. J Instit Actuaries 95:243–298

Remmen HV, Ward WF, Sabia RV, Richardson A (1995) Gene expression and protein degradation. Handbook of physiology: Section 11, Aging. Masoro EJ (ed) New York, Oxford University Press Chapter 9

Rose MR (1991) Evolutionary biology of aging. New York, Oxford University Press

Sacher GA (1956) On the statistical nature of mortality. Radiology 67:250–257

Sacher GA (1977) Life table modification and life prolongation. Handbook of the biology of aging. Finch CE, Hayflick L (eds) New York, Van Nostrand Reinhold, 582–638

Sacher GA, Trucco E (1962) The stochastic theory of mortality. Ann NY Acad Sci 96(4):985–1007

Schildkraut JM, Myers RH, Cupples LA, Kiely DK, Kannel WB (1989) Coronary risk associated with age and sex of parental heart disease in the Framingham Study. Am J Cardiol 64:555–559

Shock NW, Greulich RC, Costa PT, Andres R, Lakatta EG, Arenberg D, Tobin JD (1984) Normal human aging: the Baltimore longitudinal study of aging. NIH Publication No. 84–2450. Washington D.C., U.S. Government Printing Office

Short R, Williams DD, Bowden DM (1997) Circulating antioxidants as determinants of the rate of biological aging in pigtailed macaques. J Gerontol Biol Sci 52A(1):B25–B38

Snowdon D, Kane RL, Beeson WL, Burke GL, Sprafka JM, Potter J, Iso H, Jacobs DR, Phillips RL (1989) Is early natural menopause a biologic marker of health and aging? Am J Public Health 79(6):709–714

Sohal RS (1986) The rate of living theory: a contemporary interpretation. Insect aging: strategies and mechanisms. Collatz KG, Sohal RS (eds) Berlin, Springer-Verlag, 23–44

Strehler BL, Mildvan AS (1960) General theory and mortality of aging. Science 132:14–21

Suzman RM, Manton KG, Willis DP (1992) Introducing the oldest old. The oldest old. Willis DP, Suzman RM, Manton KG (eds) New York, Oxford University Press, 3–14

Taeuber CM, Rosenwaike I (1992) A demographic portrait of America's oldest old. The oldest old. Willis DP, Suzman RM, Manton KG (eds) New York, Oxford University Press, 17–49

Thatcher AR, Kannisto V, Vaupel JW (1998) The force of mortality at ages 80 to 120. Odense, Denmark, Odense University Press

Timiras PS (ed) (1994) Physiological basis of aging and geriatrics. Boca Raton, CRC Press.

Vaupel JW (1997) Trajectories of mortality at advanced ages. Between Zeus and the salmon: the biodemography of longevity. Wachter KW, Finch CE (eds) Washington, DC, National Academy Press

Vaupel JW, Carey JR (1993) Compositional interpretations of medfly mortality. Science 260:1666–1667

Vaupel JW, Manton KG, Stallard E (1979) The impact of heterogeneity in individual frailty on the dynamics of mortality. Demography 16(3):439–454

Vaupel JW, Johnson TE, Lithgow GJ (1994) Rates of mortality in populations of *Caenorhabditis elegans*. Science 266:826

Vaupel JW, Carey JR, Christensen K, Johnson TE, Yashin AI, Holm NV, Iachine IA, Kannisto V, Khazaeli AA, Liedo P, Longo VD, Zeng Y, Manton KG, Curtsinger JW (1998) Biodemographic trajectories of lingevity. Science 280:855–860

Yashin AI, Vaupel JW, Iachine IA (1994) A duality in aging: the equivalence of mortality models based on radically different concepts. Mech Ageing Devel 74:1–14

Resistance to Causes of Death: A Study of Cancer Mortality Resistance in the Oldest Old

D. W. E. SMITH[1]

Abstract

Very old humans do not have Gompertzian mortality rates. Their mortality rates are less than would be predicted if the mortality rate doubled at a constant rate throughout the human life span. A very small percentage of humans reach an age (<90 years) when non-Gompertzian mortality rates are seen. Cancer mortality at old age exhibits non-Gompertzian rates. Based on 1990 United States vital statistics, cancer mortality rates increase more slowly with age than mortality rates from all causes of death combined or from circulatory diseases. The mortality rates from all kinds of cancer combined and from cancer of most sites peak at 80–94 years and decline at greater ages. Individuals who reach these ages have survived the cancer and other causes of death from which the majority in their cohorts died. They are relatively resistant to cancer and other causes of death.

One can speculate about the characteristics that make these individuals relatively resistant to cancer. They include different metabolism of carcinogens, genetic factors favoring resistance, such as alleles of tumor suppressor genes and oncogenes, epigenetic factors, and less exposure to carcinogens.

Studies on identical twins suggest that environmental factors are more important than genetic factors in determining the risks of dying of cancer.

More people will survive to very old ages in the future than do today because of preventive measures and therapeutic interventions that reduce mortality rates. In order to survive, these people must be relatively resistant to dying from cancer, and some of the preventive and therapeutic interventions will be directed specifically at cancer.

The most interesting paradoxes of human longevity are those that involve non-Gompertzian mortality rates. The nineteenth century actuary Benjamin Gompertz and subsequent investigators observed that the mortality rate of humans doubles approximately every eight years of age during adult life (Finch et al. 1990). At extreme old age – over 90 years – the doubling time is longer. This finding is shown in Figure 1.

---

[1] Department of Pathology and Buehler Center on Aging. Northwestern University Medical School, 750 North Lake Shore Drive, Chicago, IL 60611-3008.

J.-M. Robine et al. (Eds.)
Research and Perspectives in Longevity
The Paradoxes of Longevity
© Springer-Verlag Berlin Heidelberg New York 1999

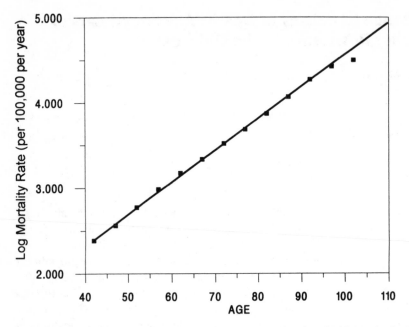

Fig. 1. Semilogarithmic plot of mortality rate against age. As first described by Benjamin Gompertz, the human mortality rate increases exponentially with age, with a doubling time of about eight years during adult life (Finch 1990), as indicated by the straight diagonal line. At great ages the rate of increase slows, as indicated by the two points at ages over 90 that fall below the line. The data are from Vital Statistics of the United States, 1990. Redrawn from Smith (1996)

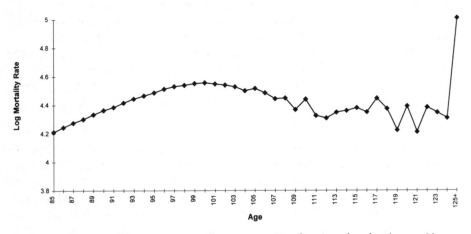

Fig. 2. Mortality rates at great ages. Log mortality rates at age 85 and over are plotted against age. Mortality rates increase to about age 90, with a doubling time of about eight years, as shown in Figure 1. At greater ages the rate of increase slows and plateaus, and mortality rates decrease beyond 105 years. Beyond 110 years mortality rates are based on very few individuals and show much scatter. Data are from United States Vital Statistics, 1956–1987. Redrawn from Riggs and Millechia (1992)

Figure 2 shows details of human mortality rates from age 85 to the maximum human life span (Riggs and Millechia 1992). The pace of increase in the mortality rats slows at about age 95, plateaus, and, for the very small number of people who reach 105 and over, the mortality rate is less than it is in younger individuals.

Although vital statistics data from the United States, on which figures 1 and 2 are based, have been criticized for showing more very old people and more deaths at extreme old age than vital statistics from other countries (Kannisto 1988), non-Gompertzian mortality rates at extreme old age are seen in the vital statistics of other developed countries (Barrett 1985; Kannisto 1988; Horiuchi and Coale 1990).

With the human species, the percentage of individuals who reach the age when non-Gompertzian mortality rates are observed is very small, and non-Gompertzian mortality rates are seen during only a small percentage of the total human life span. With some other species the percentages are greater. In the case of a large population of medflies, at least 20 % survived to an age when non-Gompertzian mortality rates were observed, and the period from this age to the maximum population life span was about 80 % of the total life span (Carey et al. 1992). We have coined the term "longevity outliers" for those individuals that live to an age when non-Gompertzian mortality rates are seen (Smith 1994).

My interpretation of lower than predicted mortality rates near the end of the life span is that the individuals that survive so long have lower mortality rates from the beginning, but only have a noticeable effect on the mortality rate of the population when most of the individuals in the population have died. Longevity outliers are themselves heterogeneous, as evidenced by their varied life spans and causes of death (Smith 1993; Olshansky 1995).

Cancer Mortality Rates

Mortality rates from cancer increase more slowly than mortality rates from all causes combined. The cancer mortality rate increases approximately linearly with age up to about 85 years, after which it plateaus and then declines, as shown in Figure 3 (Smith 1996).

These data are also based on vital statistics from the United States, which are derived from death certificate data (National Center for Health Statistics 1994). Several studies indicate that certificates that show cancer as the underlying cause of death are more accurate than death certificates showing most other causes of death (Hoel et al. 1993). There is commonly a tissue diagnosis in cancer cases.

As shown in Figure 4, mortality rates of cancer of some sites increase approximately linearly with age, and mortality rates of cancer of other sites increase more or less logarithmically with age. Mortality rates of cancer of many sites plateau and decline at very old ages, with the exception of female breast cancer (Smith 1996). With some kinds of cancer the decline is to about half of the peak mortality rates. These data, which are about mortality, and data about the clinical incidence of cancer are consistent with each other (Miller et al. 1993). The rate of

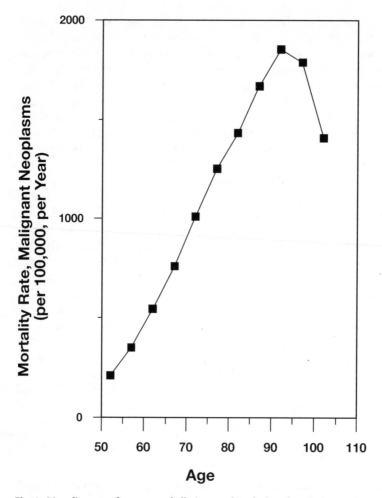

Fig. 3. Mortality rates for cancer of all sites combined plotted against age. Cancer mortality rates increase with age, but the relationship is more linear than exponential. Cancer mortality rates plateau at about 85 years and decline at ages over 90. Redrawn from Smith (1996)

incidence of cancer of several sites increases, plateaus, and declines at slightly younger ages than mortality rates. It seems reasonable that changes in incidence should precede changes in mortality.

In contrast to cancer, mortality rates from circulatory diseases, including ischemic heart disease, increase exponentially with age throughout the life span, except that the rate of increase slows slightly as 100 years is approached, as shown in Figure 5. These data are consistent with the non-Gompertzian mortality rates from all causes at ages around 100, as discussed above.

A consequence of the difference between cancer mortality rates and mortality rates from all causes combined is that cancer accounts for a progressively

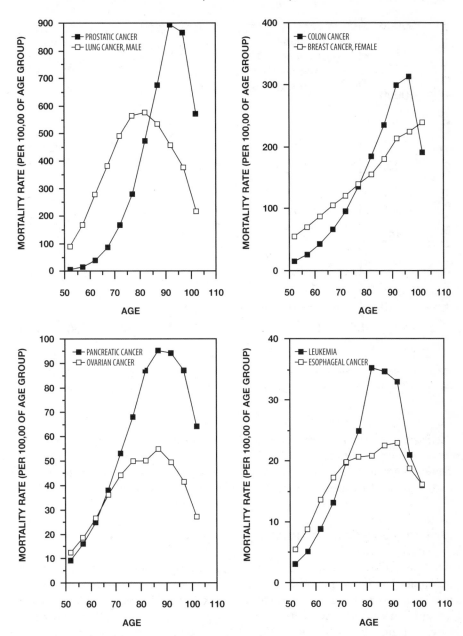

Fig. 4. Mortality rates of cancer of several sites plotted against age. Cancer Mortality rates increase, plateau, and decline with increasing age, consistent with Figure 3. Female breast cancer is an exception. Redrawn from Smith (1996)

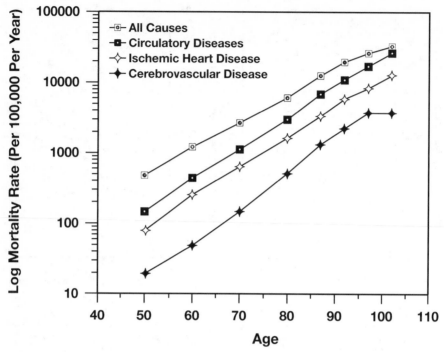

Fig. 5. Mortality rates from circulatory diseases plotted against age. In contrast to cancer, the mortality rates of circulatory diseases increase with age beyond 100 years. Redrawn from Smith (1997a)

decreasing percentage of the total deaths with age. The percentage peaks in the 50–60 age group, with nearly 40% of all deaths being attributed to cancer. The percentage is about 10% at 90–94 years and 4% over 100 years. The decline in the percentage of deaths attributed to cancer with age is shown in Figure 6 (Smith 1996).

Resistance to Cancer Mortality

What were some characteristics of the people who survive to great ages – longevity outliers, as defined above? Most in their cohort predeceased them. They do not die of cancer because of unusually low cancer mortality rates, and they do not die of other causes either. One does not become a longevity outlier with resistance to cancer but with major risk factors for dying of heart disease.

What is involved in resistance to cancer? Risk factors to cancer can be divided into exogenous risk factors and endogenous risk factors, with some having features of both. Tumorigenesis is a complex multistep process, and there is much opportunity for interaction among the risk factors.

There are genetic factors that determine susceptibility and resistance to cancer in the form of alleles of oncogenes and tumor suppressor genes. They may be

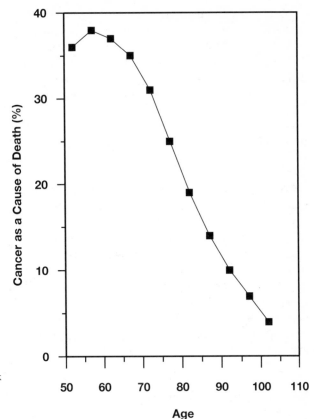

Fig. 6. Cancer mortality as a percentage of total mortality plotted against age. Cancer mortality as a percentage of total mortality reaches a peak at 50–60 and decreases at greater ages. Redrawn from Smith (1996)

inherited or result from somatic cell mutation. These alleles are recognized by their frequency of occurrence in tumors in contrast to non-neoplastic tissue. An example is p53, the product of a tumor suppressor gene. There are alleles of p53 that are characteristic of cancer (Hollstein et al. 1991).

There are epigenetic processes that could affect cancer mortality. They were discussed by Finch (1997) at the first IPSEN Fondation conference on longevity. He was considering ways to explain the heterogeneity of life spans in inbred laboratory animals kept under carefully controlled conditions – animals of nearly clonal similarity which, in spite of this genetic homogeneity, show diversity in life spans. Inbred animals also show heterogeneity in numbers of oocytes in the ovaries and of hippocampal neurons. A likely explanation is stochastic differences in the distribution of cells during development. Genetics and environment influence cell distribution, but there are stochastic differences even in the face of genetic and environmental uniformity. Finch suggested that heterogeneity of life spans in inbred laboratory animals could result from epigenetic heterogeneity in development.

There are genetic determinants of the metabolism of carcinogens, which are converted to more and less active compounds, making them, for example, more or less potent mutagens to initiate carcinogenesis.

There are genetic determinants of somatic maintenance (Kirkwood 1997) that can affect cancer resistance. There is, for example, the repair of DNA damage.

Not all cancer resistance is genetic. Except for a few tumors with well-defined genes, such as retinoblastoma and some breast cancer, there is not much familial clustering of cancer, not much concordance of cancer incidence in family members. This finding is much in contrast to diseases of the circulatory system, in which the occurrence in a parent or a sibling is a major risk factor (Goldbourt and Neufeld 1986).

Studies on identical twins have been used to separate the effects of genetics and environment on longevity. A good example is the study by Sorensen and co-workers of Danish twins separated when young and raised in different homes (Sorensen et al. 1988). There was little evidence of concordance of cancer and infectious disease deaths in the twins, but there was good evidence of coincidence of heart disease deaths.

One must look, therefore, to the environment for the major determinants of cancer mortality. Populations and individuals vary in exposure to carcinogens, such as tobacco smoke and environmental and industrial carcinogens. In addition, the significance of exposure may vary greatly according to the time in life of exposure.

Recent Changes in Mortality

Since 1950 the mean life expectancy at birth in the United States has increased from 65.6 years for males and 71.4 years for females in 1950 to 72.3 and 79.0 years, respectively, in 1994. Age adjusted mortality rates have decreased from 1,000 per 100,000 males per year and 690 per 100,000 females in 1950 to 550 and 380 per 100,000 in 1994 (Metropolitan life 1997). Most of these changes have resulted from decreased mortality rates from circulatory diseases in all age groups (Smith 1997a). Healthier lifestyles, aspirin, pacemakers, the effective control of hypertension, drugs that reduce circulating cholesterol, and coronary bypass surgery have all contributed to decreased circulatory disease mortality rates (Levy 1984). These interventions are both preventive and therapeutic. More people are living longer because of reduced mortality rates from circulatory diseases. Some people who are resistant to cancer but who would have died in the past of circulatory diseases will not do so now because of interventions. What will happen to mortality rate predictions based on Gompertz as more people live to the age of longevity outliers? Will they lave lower-than-predicted mortality rates like the longevity outliers of today? What will be their cancer mortality rates? Some who survive to advanced ages will do so with the help of interventions against circulatory disease mortality, but their survival will continue to depend on resistance to cancer mortality.

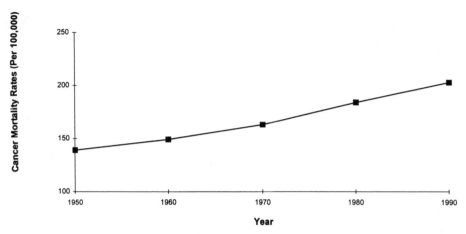

Fig. 7. Changes in cancer death rates, 1950–1990. Cancer death rates increased during the 40 year period. (National Center for Health Statistics, 1994)

Age-adjusted mortality rates for all kinds of cancer combined in all age groups and both sexes have increased 40 % in the United States between 1950 and 1990, as shown in Figure 7 (Marshall 1990; National Center for Health Statistics 1994). There is evidence based on vital statistics of the 1990s and reported recently in the popular press that this upward trend in cancer mortality rates has stopped. Cancer mortality and incidence rates may actually be decreasing (e.g., Wingo 1998).

Closer examination of cancer mortality rates during the 1980s reveals that cancer mortality rates have been declining in both males and females under 60 years of age. Admittedly, less than 15 % of all cancer deaths occurred in these younger age groups in 1990. Decreasing mortality rates in all age groups are occurring for cancer of the stomach, as shown in Figure 8. There are probably dietary reasons for this. Mortality rates are also declining for cancer of the uterine cervix and cancer of the endometrium, chiefly because of effective screening for these tumors, which allows early detection and treatment. Lung cancer mortality rates are presently falling in both males and females under 55. Fewer people are smoking, and this is resulting in reduced lung cancer mortality in younger age groups, but the effect of reduced smoking will take a long time to affect all age groups (National Center for Health Statistics 1994). So far most of the reductions in cancer mortality are due to preventive measures. One should not, however, discount the possibility of reduced cancer mortality because of therapeutic interventions. Reduced leukemia mortality rates in younger age groups are presently attributed to therapeutic interventions.

A truly interesting paradox of longevity is centenarian smokers, of whom there are a few (Franke 1997). The majority of smokers are dead by the age of 70, and for those who do not die with the majority, the mortality rate from lung cancer continues to increase to about age 85, as shown in Figure 4 (National Center for Health Statistics 1994). At still greater ages the rate declines. A few smokers,

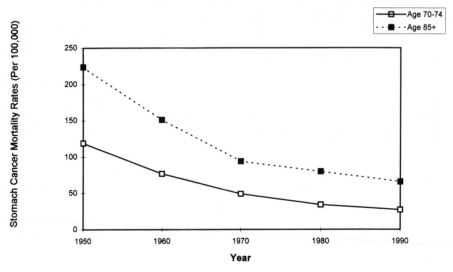

Fig. 8. Mortality rates from stomach cancer, 1950–1990. In each of two age groups, mortality rates from stomach cancer have decreased steadily during this 40 year period (National Center for Health Statistics, 1994)

however, live on and see their 100th birthdays. They must be resistant to both smoking-related cancers and smoking-related diseases of the circulatory system.

A consequence of reduced mortality rates in more very old people. There were about 30,000 people aged 100 and over in the United States as of the 1990 census (U.S. Bureau of the Census 1992). Between 1980 and 1990 the number of centenarians doubled. Assuming that this rate of increase continued through the 1990s, there may now be about 50,000 centenarians in the Unites States. There are predictions of one to two million centenarians by 2080 and scenarios of a nation expending most of its resources taking care of the very old (Vaupel and Gowan 1986). I do not think it will happen (Smith 1995). It is difficult to imagine medical advances that will sustain such a rate of growth of the centenarian population. Developed societies are now considering the need to set limits on rapidly increasing health care expenses by restricting the conditions and people on which resources should be expended. Most centenarians are in terrible condition. The mean life expectancy at age 100 is another one to two years (Smith 1997b). The chapter by Forette (1997) from the first IPSEN Conference on Longevity and some other writings on the subject (e.g., Perls 1997)), however, indicate that about one quarter of those 100 years old are in quite good condition. I think societies of the future will be less supportive of very old people in poor condition, but even if only those who are in good condition survive, there will be many more very old people than today. More people will approach today's record of human life span of 122 years set by Jeanne Calment (Robine and Allard 1995). We may expect to see her record broken; however, I believe that the human life span is approaching a limit and that the new records will exceed that of Jeanne Calment only marginally.

References

Barrett JC (1985) The mortality of centenarians in England and Wales. Arch Gerontol Geriat 4:211–218

Bureau of the Census (1992) 1990 Census of Population, General Population Characteristics, Vol. CP1-1. US Department of Commerce, Washington

Carey JR, Liendo P, Orozco D, Vaupel JW (1992) Slowing of mortality rates at older ages in large medfly cohorts. Science 258:457–461

Finch CE (1997) Longevity: Is everything under genetic control? An inquiry into non-genetic and non-environmental sources of variation. In: Robine J-M, Vaupel JW, Jeune B, Allard M (eds) Longevity: To the limits and beyond. Springer Verlag, Berlin, pp. 167–178

Finch CE, Pike M, Whitten M (1990) Slow mortality rate accelerations during aging in some animals approximate that in humans. Science 249:902–905

Forette B (1997) Centenarians: health and frailty. In: Robine J-M, Vaupel JW, Jeune B, Allard M (eds) Longevity: To the limits and beyond. Springer Verlag, Berlin, pp. 105–112

Franke H (1997) New special research on over 100 year old probands. Zeits Gerontol Geriat 30:130–155

Goldbourt U, Neufeld HN (1986) Genetic aspects of atherosclerosis. Atherosclerosis 6:357–377

Hoel DG, Ron E, Carter R, Mabuchi K (1993) Influence of death certificate errors on Cancer mortality statistics. J Nat Cancer Inst 85:1063–1066

Hollstein M, Sidransky D, Vogelstein B, Harris CC (1991) p53 mutations in human cancers. Science 253:49–53

Horiuchi S, Coale AL (1990) Mortality of older women: An analysis using age-specific rate of mortality change with age. Math Pop Stud 2:245–267

Kannisto V (1988) On the survival of centenarians and the span of life. Pop Stud 42:389–406

Kirkwood TBL (1997) Human senescence. BioEssays 18:1009–1016

Levy RI (1984) Causes of the decrease in cardiovascular mortality. Am J Cardiol 51 (supplement): 7C–13C

Marshall E (1990) Experts clash over cancer data. Science 250:900–902

Metropolitan Life (1997) Record high U.S. life expectancy. Statistical Bulletin 78(4):2–8

Miller BA, Ries LSG, Hankey BF, Cosary CL, Harrass A, Devesa SS, Edwards EK (1993) SEER Cancer Statistical Review, 1973–1990 (Publication No. 93-2789). National Institutes of Health, Bethesda

National Center for Health Statistics (1994) Vital Statistics of the United States, Vol II, part A. US Public Health Service, Washington. (And other years as shown)

Olshansky SJ (1995) Introduction: New developments in mortality. Gerontologist 35:583–587

Perls T (1997) Genetic determinants of longevity. Gerontologist 37. Special Issue: 47

Riggs JE, Millechia D (1992) Mortality among the elderly in the U.S., 1956–1987: Demonstration of the upper boundary to Gompertzian mortality. Mech Ageing Devel 62:191–199

Robine JM, Allard M (1995) Validation of the exceptional longevity case of a 120 years old woman. Facts Res Gerontol 363–367

Wingo PA, Ries LAG, Rosenberg HM, Miller DS, Edwards BK. Cancer incidence and Mortality, 1973–1995. Cancer 1998; 82:197–207

Smith DWE (1995) Why do we live so long? Omega 31:143–150

Smith DWE (1993) Human longevity. Oxford University Press, New York

Smith DWE (1994) The tails of survival curves. BioEssays 16:907–911

Smith DWE (1996) Cancer mortality at very old ages. Cancer 77:1367–1372

Smith DWE (1997a) Circulatory disease mortality in the very elderly. Epidemiology 8:50

Smith DWE (1997b) Centenarians: Longevity outliers. Gerontologist 37:200–207

Sorensen TIA, Nielsen GG, Andersen PK, Teasdale TW (1988) Genetic and environmental differences on premature death in adult adoptees. New Engl J Med 318:727–732

Vaupel JW, Gowan AE (1986) Passage to Methuselah: Some demographic consequences of continued progress against mortality. Am J Public Health 76:430–433

Are Common Risk Factors Relevant in the Eldest Old?

B. FORETTE[1]

The recent growth of the eldest segment of the population has made possible studies that were unimaginable or meaningless some decades ago. At the beginning of the century, who would have considered drawing up a centenarians' life expectancy table? Assessing risk factors for mortality and morbidity in very old people is now a necessity, and we progressively discover some amazing differences from the well-established results in younger persons. Several major risk factors do not seem to play the same role at a very old age, and the relationship between mortality and some classic risk factors may even appear to be reversed. Among those risk factors are male gender, body weight, high blood pressure and total serum cholestrol.

Gender

Being a man is obviously a strong risk factor for mortality until an advanced age. Men seem to be more sensitive to a large variety of pathogenic conditions. Among centenarians, the male/female ratio was 1/7 in the IPSEN survey (Forette 1997). However, in all studies, male centenarians have a better general health status and achieve higher cognitive performances than women. Cardiovascular diseases become more prevalent in centenarian women than in men (Beregi et al. 1995). Male centenarians have better capacities than female, they need less assistance, they have more teeth of their own, and their sight and hearing are better.

In the IPSEN study, more men than women were able to be tested with the Pfeiffer's Short Portable Questionnaire, and the mean score of men was significantly better. Dementia was significantly more frequent in women than in men: about one of two vs. one of five in the French, Hungarian and Finnish studies (Allard 1991; Ivan 1990; Louhija 1994). Male centenarians have significantly better language ability, social integration, orientation, sphincter continence, physical independence and mobility than female centenarians. Is the male advantage in very old age due to a stronger selection, leaving only a small "biological elite" in late life, or does male gender confer some kind of resistance to specific alterations induced by extreme aging?

[1] Centre Claude Bernard de Gérontologie, Hôpital Sainte Périne, 11, Rue Chardon-Lagache, 75781 Paris, France.

J.-M. Robine et al. (Eds.)
Research and Perspectives in Longevity
The Paradoxes of Longevity
© Springer-Verlag Berlin Heidelberg New York 1999

Body Weight

Body weight is a well-established risk factor in adults under 65, but not in the elderly. In a three-year prospective study of 722 persons aged 84–82 years, living in their own homes in the city of Tampere (Finland), mortality was not increased in those with body-mass $\geq 30\,kg/m^2$ (Rajala et al. 1990). Recent data from the Framingham study confirm that excess body weight increases the risk of death from any cause and from cardiovascular disease in adults between 30 and 74 years of age (Stevens et al. 1998). The relative risk asssociated with an increase in the body-mass index declines with age among men and women for both mortality from all causes and mortality from cardiovascular disease (Larson 1995). For subjects over 85 years old, the relative risk associated with an increment of 1.0 in body-mass index is either zero (men) or negative (women) after adjustment for age, education, physical activity and alcohol consumption. Potential confounding factors have to be more carefully examined in older subjects, who may have weight reduction because of associated illness. However, the fact that risk does not increase at lower body-mass index in older subjects argues against this possibility (Stevens et al. 1998).

Blood Pressure

The early reports from the Framingham study showed that high blood pressure was a risk factor for cardiovascular diseases until the age of 74 (Dawber et al. 1957). Several randomized trials have demonstrated a benefit of treatment in hypertensive patients over 60 years old, but the results are less clear above 80 years (Staessen et al. 1989; Dahlöf et al. 1991; SHEP 1991).

A positive association between high blood pressure and survival in very old people was found ten years ago in a Finnish cohort (Mattila et al. 1988). In the city of Tampere, 83 % of the citizens aged 85 or more (561 persons) were divided into six groups on the basis of their blood pressure. Their mean age was 88.4 ± 2.8 years, more than half were living at home, and 82 % were women. The cohort was followed-up for five years; age and gender were taken into account to estimate relative survival rates. The mortality was highest in the lowest systolic and lowest diastolic blood pressure groups. Better survival was observed in the groups with systolic pressures of 160 mm Hg and over, and with diastolic pressures of 90 mm Hg and over. The five-year survival rate (59 %) of patients with hypertensive disease was significantly higher than the survival rate of the other groups (28 %). Moreover, the survival rate of patients in the highest systolic hypertensive group (>200 mm Hg) was significantly better than the survival rate of the "normotensive" (140–159 mm Hg) group.

These surprising results were confirmed in other studies, especially in men (Langer et al. 1989). Yet several criticisms have been made of the association between elevated pressure and reduced cardiovascular as well as all-cause mortality. Low blood pressure may be the result of underlying illness. In a population of 3657 elderly residents of East Boston, higher systolic pressure predicted linear increases in cardiovascular and total mortality after adjustment for confounding variables (including frailty and disorders such as congestive heart failure and myocardial infarction) and exclusion of deaths within the first three years of the 10.5 year follow-up. After the same adjustments, higher diastolic pressure predicted a linear increase in cardiovascular mortality but not total mortality (Taylor et al. 1991; Glynn et al. 1995). In the Framingham study, subjects over 75 were divided into two groups (Kannel and D'Agostino 1997). In those with cardiovascular disease at the biennial examination there was a distinct U-shaped curve of cardiovascular mortality rate in relation to systolic blood pressure in men, with a substantial increase in mortality rate below systolic pressure of 120 mm Hg for both men and women. In the sample of subjects free of cardiovascular disease there were increasing cardiovascular morbidity and mortality rates with increasing blood pressure levels for both men and women. The conclusion was that the excess mortality rate reported for low blood pressure levels in persons older than 75 years derives from the inclusion of the substantial proportion of this age group who have cardiovascular disease.

These criticisms, however, are not totally convincing. The population that they are based on is not strictly limited to the old-old. To explore the possible reasons of the paradoxical survival of hypertensive elderly, all-cause mortality and cardiovascular mortality were analyzed in 795 persons aged 75–96 and followed prospectively for three years in the Rancho Bernardo Chronic Disease Study (Langer et al. 1991). Survival analyses showed a significant trend for improved survival, with increasing diastolic pressure in men aged 80 years and older versus all-cause mortality and cardiovascular mortality. Results were not explained by a wide range of biological and historical factors: differences in the use of antihypertensive medication, pulse pressure, history of hypertension, history of coronary heart disease, isolated systolic hypertension, interval change in diastolic pressure over an average of 12 years, or by cholesterol, triglycerides, fasting plasma glucose, smoking, or body mass index.

In conclusion: a positive relationship between survival and high blood pressure has been demonstrated in subjects aged 85 years and over. To date, the role of potential confounding factors that might explain this relationship has not been proved in populations of strictly comparable age.

Cholesterol

Total serum cholesterol values tend to rise during life, but not beyond age 60 in men and 70 in women. Concentrations then decrease slightly. This trend has been observed in cross-sectional as well as longitudinal studies (Ettinger et al. 1992).

As a cardiovascular risk factor, serum cholesterol cencentration becomes less important with increasing age, and eventually disappears in the oldest old. In a study of 2544 men undergoing coronary angiography, the association between plasma cholesterol and severity of coronary occlusion held only for the younger men, diminishing to near zero in the oldest age group (Jacobsen et al. 1992). Moreover, almost all studies in very old people show that low plasma cholesterol levels are related to an elevated total mortality, and this phenomenon cannot be totally explained by the usual confounding factors. We followed-up for five years a group of elderly women (mean age, 82.2) living in a nursing fome (Forette et al. 1989). Mortality was lowest at serum cholesterol 7.0 mmol/L, 5.2 times higher when cholesterol concentration was 8.8 mmol/L, and only 1.8 times higher than the minimum when cholesterol concentration was 8.8 mmol/L. This relation held true even when blood pressure, body weight, history of myocardial infarction, creatinine clearance and plasma proteins were taken into account. The relation between low cholesterol values and increased mortality was independent of the incidence of cancer. We repeated the study in another group of elderly women (mean age, 89.9) followed-up for seven years. We found again a reversed J-shaped relation between serum total cholesterol and mortality. Mortality was lowest at serum cholesterol 7.2 mmol/1, 5.5 times higher than the minimum at serum cholesterol 2.9 mmol/l and only 1.5 higher when total cholesterol concentration was 9.3 mmol/l. We did not found any significant relationship between mortality and HDL cholesterol. Mortality was also independent of total/HDL cholesterol ratio.

In the Framingham study (Kronmal et al. 1993), the relationship between total cholesterol level and all-cause mortality was positive (higher cholesterol level associated with higher mortality) at age 40 years, negligible at ages 50 to 70 years, and significantly negative at age 80 years (higher cholesterol level associated with lower mortality). The relationship of total cholesterol with coronary heart disease (CHD) mortality was significantly positive at ages 40 to 60 (but decreasing with age), not significant at age 70 years, and negative (but not significant) at age 80 years. Non-CHD mortality was significantly negatively related to cholesterol level for ages 50 years and above.

Similar results were observed in a ten-year Dutch study including 724 participants whose median age was 89 years. High total cholesterol concentrations were associated with longevity, owing to lower mortality from cancer and infections, whereas cardiovascular mortality was independent of cholesterol level (Weverling-Rijnsburger et al. 1997).

Some data suggest that low cholesterol might impair brain functions (Mason et al. 1991; Svennerholm et al. 1994). An excess of violent deaths has been reported when serum cholesterol of middle aged patients was lowered with diet, drugs, or both in primary cardiovascular prevention trials (Muldoon et al. 1990). Low cholesterol levels have been shown to possibly slow mental processing (Benton 1995) and to be linked with depressive symptoms in older men (Morgan et al. 1993; Brown et al. 1994). As very old people seem more susceptible to adverse effects of hypocholesterolemia, we tried to test the relation between serum cholesterol and cognitive performance in a population drawn from the nationwide survey of French centenarians conducted for one year by the IPSEN Foundation. We selected 107 centenarian women (mean age, 101.8 years; range, 100.0 to 115.4) who were not bedribben and who were able to complete the Pfeif-

Table 1. Cholesterol and Pfeiffer's test (107 non-bedridden women centenarians)

Cholesterol (mmol/L)	2.9–5.0	5.1–6.0	6.1–8.0
Subjects	39	33	35
Number of errors (SD)	4.6 (3.1)	3.5 (3.0)	2.6 (2.2)
p <0,01 (ANOVA)			

fer's Short Portable Mental Status Questionnaire (SPMSQ), which only takes a few minutes and may be passed by people with mild sensory impairment (Pfeiffer 1975). There was a significant negative relationship between serum cholesterol concentration and the number of errors in the SPMSQ ($r = -0.25$, $p <0.01$). It is interesting to note that centenarian women whose serum cholesterol levels were in the pathological range performed better (i.e., made less errors) than those who had normal cholesterol values (Table 1). When taking serum albumin into account, a linear negative relationship remained between cholesterol and the number of errors in SPMSQ ($r = -0.32$, $p <0.05$). These data suggest that cognitive functions of centenarians may be positively related to blood cholesterol, and that this relationship is not explained solely by a better general nutritional status in subject with higher cholesterol level.

Change in the impact of some risk factors in the oldest old is a very controversial issue since, with increasing age, confounding factors become both more numerous and less easy to detect. For example, low blood pressure may be the consequence of many cardiovascular diseases. It has been argued that lower cholesterol may result from underlying diseases such as cancer, infection, or any cause of poor nutrition. But several studies suggest that the paradox holds true even when these factors are adjusted for. The Established Populations for Epidemiologic Studies in the Elderly (EPESE) was supposed to clarify the direct relationship between total cholesterol levels and death from coronary heart disease in older persons (Corti et al. 1997). In that five-year prospective study, total cholesterol was negatively related to coronary heart disease. The relationship became positive only after adjustment for over 14 factors and exclusion of deaths from coronary heart disease which occurred within the first year. Moreover, the mean age of the participants was only 79 years. Similar limitations can apply to other studies intended to demonstrate that cholesterol remains a risk factor for mortality in advanced age.

Thus, all of the paradoxical changes observed at a very old age in the role of some major risk factors do not appear to be totally explained. People who are able to live more than 85 or 90 years may differ in several ways from those who die earlier; they should be considered separately inside the populations of "65 years and over." The need for special studies of risk factors in the oldest old appears especially urgent since the fastest growing segment of the population is people ages 85 years and over.

References

Allard M (1991) A la recherche du secret des centenaires. Le Cherche-Midi, Paris

Benton D (1995) Do low cholesterol levels show mental processing? Psychosom Med 57:50–53

Beregi E, Regius O, Nemeth J, Rajczy K, Gergely I, Lengyel E (1995) Gender differences in age-related physiological changes and some diseases. Z Gerontol Geriatr 28:62–66

Brown SL, Salive ME, Harris TB, Simonsick EM, Guralnik JM, Kohout FJ (1994) Low cholesterol concentration and severe depressive symptoms in elderly people. Br Med J 308: 1328–1332

Corti MC, Guralnik JM, Salive ME, Harris T, Ferrucci L, Glynn R, Havlik RJ (1997) Clarifying the direct relation between total cholesterol levels and death from coronary heart disease in older persons. Ann Intern Med 126:753–760

Dahlöf B, Lindholm LH, Hansson L, Scherstén B, Ekbom T, Wester PO (1991) Morbidity and mortality in the Swedish Trial in Old Patients with Hypertension (STOP-Hypertension). Lancet 338:1281–1285

Dawber TR, Moore FE, Mann GV (1957) Coronary heart disease in the Framingham study. Am J Public Health 47:25–32

Ettinger WH, Wahl PW, Kuller HL, Bush TL, Tracy RP, Manolio TA, Borhani NO, Wong ND, O'Leary DH (1992) Lipoprotein lipids in older people. Results from the cardiovascular health study. Circulation 86:858–869

Forette B (1997) Centenarians: health and frailty. In: Robine JM, Vaupel JW, Jeune B, Allard M (eds) Longevity: to the limits and beyond. Berlin Heidelberg New York, Springer Verlag 105–112

Forette B, Tortrat D, Wolmark Y (1989) Cholesterol as risk factor for mortality in elderly women. Lancet i:868–870

Glynn RJ, Fields TS, Rosner B, Hebert PR, Taylor JO, Hennekens CH (1995) Evidence for a positive linear relation between blood pressure and mortality in elderly people. Lancet 345:825–829

Ivan L (1990) Neuropsychiatric examination of centenarians. In: Beregi E (ed) Centenarians in Hungary. A social and demographic study. Interdisciplinary topics in gerontology. Vol. 27. Karger, Basel, 53–64

Jacobsen SJ, Freedman DC, Hoffmann RG, Gruchow HW, Anderson AJ, Barboriak JJ (1992) Cholesterol and coronary artery disease: age as an effect modifier. J Clin Epidemiol 45:1053–1059

Kannel WB, D'Agostino RB (1997) Blood pressure and cardiovascular morbidity and mortality rates in the elderly. Am Heart J 134:758–763

Kronmal AR, Cain KC, Ye Z, Omenn GS (1993) Total serum cholesterol levels and mortality risk as a function of age. A report based on the Framingham data. Arch Intern Med 153:1065–1073

Langer RD, Ganiats TG, Barrett-Connor E (1989) Paradoxical survival of elderly men with high blood pressure. Br Med J 298:1356–1358

Langer RD, Ganiats TG, Barrett-Connor E (1991) Factors associated with paradoxical survival at higher blood pressures in the very old. Am J Epidemiol 134:29–38

Larson MG (1995) Assessment of cardiovascular risk factors in the elderly: the Framingham Heart Study. Stat Med 14:1745–1756

Louhija (1994) Finnish centenarians. Academic dissertation, University of Helsinki

Mason RP, Herbette LG, Silverman DI (1991) Can altering serum cholesterol affect neurologic function? J Mol Cell Cardiol 23:1339–1342

Mattila K, Haaviston M, Rajala S, Heikinheimio R (1988) Blood pressure and five year survival in the very old. Br Med J 296:887–889

Morgan RE, Palinkas LA, Barrett-Connor EL, Wingard DL (1993) Plasma cholesterol and depressive symptoms in older men. Lancet 341:75–79

Muldoon MF, Manuck SB, Mathews KA (1990) Lowering cholesterol concentration and mortality: a quantitative review of primary prevention trials. Br Med J 301:309–314

Pfeiffer E (1975) A short portable mental status questionnaire for the assessment of organic brain deficit in elderly patients. J Am Geriatric Soc 23:433–445

Rajala SA, Kanto AJ, Haavisto MV, Kaarela RH, Koivunen MJ, Heikinheimo RJ (1990) Body weight and the three-year prognosis in very old people. Int J Obesity 14:997–1003

SHEP Cooperative Research Group (1991) Prevention of stroke by antihypertensive drug treatment in older persons with isolated systolic hypertension. JAMA 265:3255–3264

Staessen J, Bulpitt C, Clement D, De Leeuw P, Fagard R, Fletcher A, Forette F, Leonetti G, Nissinen A, O'Malley K, Tuomilehto J, Webster J, Williams BO (1989) Relation between mortality and treated blood pressure in elderly patients with hypertension: report of the European Working Party on High Blood Pressure in the Elderly. BMJ 298:1552–1556

Stevens J, Jianwen C, Pamuk ER, Williamson DF, Thun MJ, Wood JL (1998) The effect of age on the association between body-mass index and mortality. N Engl J Med 338:1–7

Svennerholm L, Bostrom K, Jungbjer B, Olsson L (1994) Membrane lipids of adult human brain: Lipid composition of frontal and temporal lobe in subjects of age 20 to 100 years. J Neurochem 63: 1802–1811

Taylor JO, Cornorni-Huntley J, Curb JD, Manton KG, Ostfeld AM, Scherr P, Wallace RB (1991) Blood pressure and mortality risk in the elderly. Am J Epidemiol 134:489–501

Weverling-Rijnsburger AWE, Blauw G, Lagaay AM, Knook DL, Meinders AE, Westendorp RGJ (1997) Total cholesterol and risk of mortality in the oldest old. Lancet 350:1119–11123

The "French Paradox": Nutrition and Longevity

M. Gerber[1]

Summary

The assumption that nutrition influences longevity was generated by ecological studies showing that longevity differs among countries with different patterns of food intake. Although these countries may vary in ways other than nutrition, just the knowledge that nutrition is associated with chronic degenerative diseases supports the above hypothesis. Cardiovascular diseases and cancers are the leading causes of a shortened life expectancy for the 45 to 70 age group in Western societies. Therefore, factors influencing these pathologies will affect longevity. The net effect is reinforced because most of the efficient nutrients affect both types of diseases – coronary heart diseases (CHD) and some of the most prevalent cancers (colon, breast, lung) – in the same way, although by different mechanisms. Energy-rich diets resulting in energy imbalance and a high intake of saturated fatty acids are risk factors for CHD and cancer, whereas fruit and vegetables appear to be protective or risk-reducing factors, even when the responsible nutrients are not fully identified: fiber, antioxidants, and/or other microcomponents of fruit and vegetables.

An increasing number of reports tend to demonstrate that nutrition also has an effect on ageing, and especially on cognitive functions, which might ultimately modify longevity.

France has become famous by claiming a lower mortality rate than other Western countries, in spite of food habits that are comparable in amounts of lipids and energy. The observation of lower CHD mortality rates in France compared with other Western countries, even though fat intake was estimated to be in the mid-range of the distribution across these countries, led to the concept of the "French paradox". France deviated from the regular North-South gradient. Then, the Monica study provided results based on incidence which reintegrated France in the North-South gradient. The relationship between cholesterol fat and cardiovascular disease does not encompass all the factors explaining CHD mortality. In each region, the whole food pattern must be analysed, uncluding the specific fatty acids making up the total fat intake, in the one hand cereal, fruit and vegetal intake, and fibre and antioxidants on the other hand. Also, not only

[1] Groupe d'Epidémiologie Métabolique, Centre de Recherche en Cancérologie, INSERM-CRLC, 34298 Montpellier Cedex 5, France.

J.-M. Robine et al. (Eds.)
Research and Perspectives in Longevity
The Paradoxes of Longevity
© Springer-Verlag Berlin Heidelberg New York 1999

plasma total cholesterol but also LDL- and HDL-cholesterol should be considered. By taking all of these parameters into account the French paradox, as usually proposed, vanishes.

Introduction

Human beings have always looked for a magic food in their diet which would make them centenarians: first yoghourt, then apples, and now olive oil and purslane in their salad. Epidemiological studies have shown that the prevalence of some diseases that are responsible for a shortened life span could be reduced through nutrition.

A favourable diet close to the Mediterranean diet appears to be the best way to reduce the risk of chronic degenerative diseases and especially coronary heart disease (CHD); (Kushi et al. 1995; Corpet and Gerber 1997; Gerber and Corpet 1997). Another aspect to consider is how nutrition can help us live beyond the age at risk for these diseases.

Aside from the remarkable longevity of French women, the concept of the "French paradox" was developed because the low mortality due to CHD did not fit with the total fat intake. But fat intake and cholesterolemia do not fully explain CHD. As usual, there is no one simple answer to the complexity of degenerative diseases, and taking into consideration the epidemiological bias and the various risk factors will help us to understand a large part of the "paradox."

All these aspects will be developed and illustrated below. In conclusion, I will pinpoint areas that are not yet well understood and require further research.

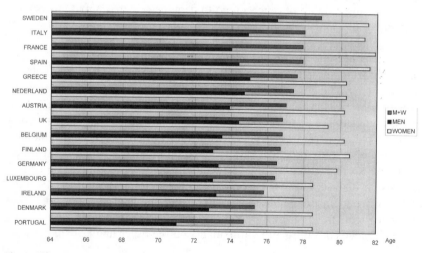

Fig. 1. Life expectancy at birth in European countries (1996)

Patterns of Life Expectancy, Food Consumption and Diseases

The assumption that nutrition influences longevity was generated by ecological studies showing that longevity differs among countries with different patterns of food intake. This finding is true when considering life expectancy at birth (Fig. 1), where Italy, Spain, France and Greece are only surpassed by Sweden, but also when considering life expectancy at age 65 (Fig. 2), which is more significant with regard to the effect on events late in life. Since malnutrition in terms of severe deficiencies has largely disappeared from the Westernized world, nutrition, either as risk factor or protective factor, is associated with chronic degenerative diseases, which are the leading causes or mortality for the 45 to 70 ages

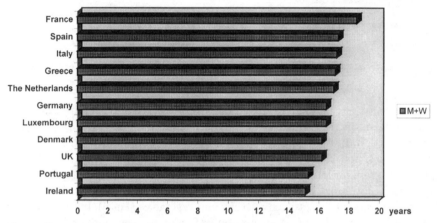

Fig. 2. Life expectancy at age 65 in European countries (1990)

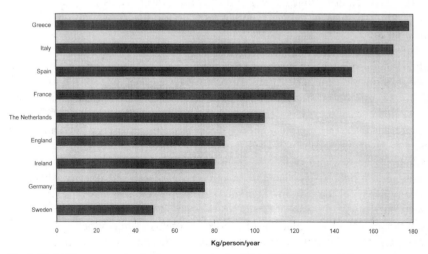

Fig. 3. Vegetable consumption in European countries 1986–1987 (Eurostat 1989)

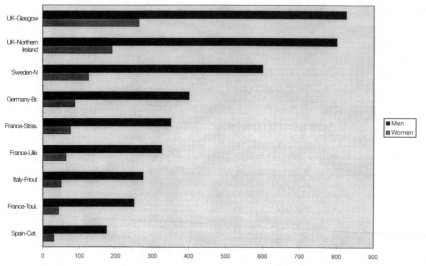

Fig. 4. Coronary heart diseases rates per 100,000 in European countries as defined in WHO MONICA (1994)

group. Seventy percent of all deaths in the group aged 65 and over are caused by cardiovascular diseases and cancers in European countries (Report from the Commission on the State of Health in the European Community, 1996).

If we look now at food consumption, the same countries who are at the top of the histogram for longevity are at the top of the histograms depicting the consumption of food that is associated with a reduction in risk for cardiovascular diseases and some cancers, such as fruits and vegetables (Fig. 3). By contrast, the situation is reversed for the consumption of food associated with an increase in risk for CHD and food-related cancers. Consequently, incidence rates of CHDs (Fig. 4; WHO Monica Project 1994) and of some cancers (Figs. 5, 6; Gerber and Corpet 1997) display a pattern similar to that for the consumption of risk-associated food.

Thus, these ecological studies suggest that nutrition affects longevity indirectly through its effect on diseases responsible for a shortened life. Of course, a causal relationship cannot be inferred from this type of comparison. But if we do not yet have etiological studies for the relationship between longevity and nutrition, we do have solid evidence showing that food habits affect the risk of chronic degenerative diseases. Too much energy intake resulting in energy imbalance and obesity is associated with increased mortality (Møller et al. 1994), both by cardiovascular diseases and cancer. A certain type of obesity is especially at risk: visceral/abdominal obesity, also named apple-type, or android, obesity. This type of obesity is part of the insulin-resistance syndrome that is a determinant of cardiovascular disease but also of hormono-dependent cancers and possibly colon cancer through the dysregulation of binding proteins of hormones and growth factors (IGF-1); (Stoll 1994; Gerber et al. 1996). Thus any excess of macronutrients might result in an excess of energy intake, but lipids, which are the most

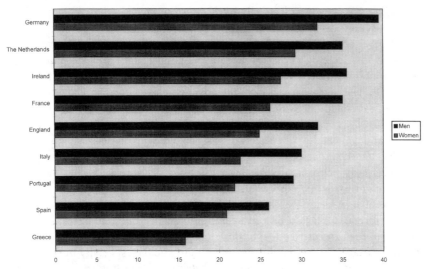

Fig. 5. Colorectal cancer incidence per 100,000 in European countries (Facts and Figures of Cancer in Europe, IARC 1993)

calorigenic but also more easily stored in adipous tissue, are generally more likely to cause obesity than carbohydrates, which are oxidized in the first place (Flatt 1995). However, an excess of carbohydrates in the absence of physical exercise will also be responsible for weight gain and might become a risk factor (Franceschi et al. 1996).

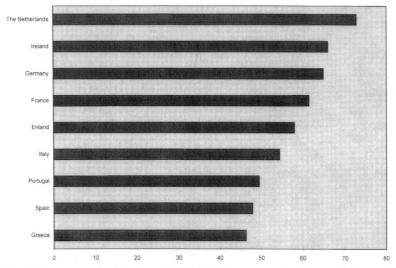

Fig. 6. Breast cancer incidence per 100,000 in European countries (Facts and Figures of Cancer in Europe, IARC 1993)

Lipids are not only quantitatively hazardous but also qualitatively, especially for cardiovascular diseases; short-chain saturated fatty acids (Yu et al. 1995) increase LDL-cholesterol more than stearic acid (18 carbon atoms). Polyunsaturated fatty acids decrease cholesterol, both the good (HDL) and the bad (LDL), whereas monounsaturated fat appers to be neutral towards LDL but tends to increase HDL. Fish and seafood have the advantage over meat in providing protein without saturated fat, even providing especially valuable polyunsaturated fat (serie n-3).

Fruits and vegetables are regularly associated with a decrease in risk in chronic degenerative diseases. In fruits and vegetables, two types of nutrient play a role in decreasing chronic degenerative disease risk: fibre and micronutrients, among them antioxidants. Fibre is also found in cereals. Fibre opposes the effect of lipids because it decreases nutrient density. Soluble fibre favors cholesterol excretion. Fibre also plays a role in keeping down insulinemia. Several mechanisms explain the protective effect of fibre in colon cancers: effect on transit time and the anticarcinogenic effect of short chain fatty acids, especially butyric acid. In the case of breast cancer, fibre may be protective because it affects the colon flora that play a role in estrogen excretion or reabsorption (Gerber 1996).

A large body of literature has been devoted to the effect of antioxidants, with observational epidemiological and animal studies being more convincing than intervention studies. For cardiovascular diseases, mainly vitamin E and, to a lesser extent, beta-carotene and vitamin C appear to be the candidates to explain this effect (reviewed in Diaz et al. 1997). These antioxidants could oppose the involvement of highly oxidized LDL in the rupture of the atherome plaque, vasoconstriction and thrombosis (Diaz et al. 1997). Vitamin C is most often found to be protective in stomach cancer. Betacarotene is the antioxidant that is most consistently associated with lung cancer and cancers of the upper respiratory and digestive tracts. However, so far there is no definitive evidence that beta-carotene is responsible for the protective effect and not another component of the vegetables. Many other components are indeed present in fruits and vegetables, such as folates, flavones and flavonoids, glucosinolates and isothiocyanates. All have recently been shown to be protective both for cardiovascular diseases and cancer (Hertog et al. 1993; Knekt et al. 1997).

So far, the same nutriments are either protective or deleterious for both CHD and cancers, which makes this effect visible on total, mortality. However, a discrepancy exists for alcohol. Alcohol consumption is associated with lower mortality by CHD, through a beneficial effect on HDL cholesterol, and a reduced thrombose risk; however, alcohol is a risk factor for cancers of the upper digestive tract, stomach and colon-rectum, and of breast in women, even at moderate doses. Alcohol might also favor obesity, and beer would be more likely to induce abdominal obesity than wine (Duncan et al. 1995).

Nutrition and Health of the Oldest Old

Before pursuing the effects of alcohol and wine – which is a natural link to the last part of this presentation, a discussion of the French paradox – some data on nutrition of the elderly are worthy of attention.

We know that a diet rich in cereals, fruits and vegetables, with a moderate intake of fat, (preferably monounsaturated fat), and a very moderate intake of wine will help to overcome these chronic degenerative diseases that are mainly responsible for a shortened life span (between 55 and 75 years). However, after one has survived these hazaradous years is the diet supposed to stay the same, to ensure longevity, or are new needs appearing?

One of the main points of discussion has been weight loss. The problem of adverse health conditions causing weight loss is likely to increase with age and to be severe in older groups because of loss of lean mass at these ages. This phenomenon probably accounts for the apparently increasing ideal weight with age in simplistic analyses relating body weight to mortality (Willett 1997). Weight stability is associated with better health status, and overweight old persons are encouraged to pursue regular physical exercise and modest weight loss. A decrease in physical activity as well as low initial levels of physical activity are strong risk factors for mortality in women aged 60 to 80 years (Lissner et al. 1996).

The same type of diet, one rich in fruits and vegetables, seems to also be beneficial not only in improving the general health of the elderly but also in improving cognitive functions (Ortega et al. 1997). Again the relative importance of carbohydrate intake versus fat intake is stressed (Ortega et al. 1997). Among the plant foods, folate appeared to be associated with cognitive functions, whereas in another study vitamin C and beta-carotene plasma levels were associated with the performance in specific tests of cognitive function (Perrig et al. 1997). Among minerals, zinc and iron intake was higher in persons with the best performance.

Finally, diversity of food appears most important. An index summarizing the various components of a diet is a better predictor of death rate than an analysis based on a single nutrient (Nube et al. 1987; Kant et al. 1993).

The French Paradox and Coronary Heart Disease

This term has been coined to account for the contradiction between the CHD mortality in France (the second lowest after Japan) and the fat intake of the French (comparable to that of countries with higher CDH mortality rate, 38–42 % of energy as fat). However, Ducimetierre and Richard (1992) were the first to suggest that the lower-than-expected CHD mortality in France may have no counterparts in terms of incidence. The results of the MONICA study (1994), based on incidence rates of acute coronary episodes, showed that France did not deviate from the North-South gradient. A bias in reporting causes of death may be an explanation, since in France the rate of "undefined causes of death"

Table 1. Mortality in France and neighbouring countries[a]

Mortality	German + Belgium		France		Italy + Spain	
	Men	Women	Men	Women	Men	Women
CHD	226	54	130	24	170	31
Cardiovascular disease	548	213	402	130	452	191
Cancers	384	252	490	206	382	193
Undefined	**39**	**16**	**49**	**16**	**15**	**5**
Other	296	138	379	150	301	120

[a] 100,000 subjects, aged 45–64.

is higher than in other European countries and can contain sudden death possibly due to cardiovascular diseases (Table 1; Ducimetierre 1995).

Another question to discuss is the relationship between the cholesterol saturated fat index and CHD mortality. When this relationship is studied in 17 countries with available wine data consumption, the correlation was high and significant (r = 0.73). France and Switzerland showed the greatest deviation from the regression line, despite above average dairy fat intake (Renaud and de Lorgeril 1992). Adjustment for the inverse effect of wine consumption moved France and Switzerland back close to the regression line, improving the correlation to r = 0.87. But in another multicentric study (Artaud-Wild et al. 1993), Finland had a higher-than-expected CHD mortality rate and France had a lower-than-expected CHD mortality rate. Lower dairy food and higher vegetable consumption partly explained this discrepancy, showing that other characteristics of the Mediterranean diet, such as vegetable, fruit and fish (Corpet and Gerber 1997) consumption, are equally important in explaining this lower-than-expected CHD mortality rate. And, indeed, various Mediteranean countries have claimed their own paradoxes; the Spanish paradox (Serra-Majem et al. 1995) and the Albanian paradox (Gjonça and Bobak, 1997). Some have also reported on the European paradox (Bellizzi et al. 1994). Criqui and Ringel (1994) analysed data from 21 countries, evaluating dietary components and alcoholic beverage as predictive of CHD and total mortality. They conclude that the "French paradox appears soluble". First, the evidence of the benefit wine over ethanol is rather weak, mostly when studied in cohorts. Indeed, when comparing the correlations of CHD mortality with wine consumption and of CHD with ethanol from wine consumption, the latter is always stays higher. This finding suggests that the possible effect of wine, independent from alcohol and due to the antioxidant capacity of the phenolic compounds of wine, is small compared to the effect of alcohol via the HDL-pathway and of effects on thrombotic factors, platelet aggregation and fibrinogen.

Thus the apparent greater benefit of wine might be an artefact. Consumption of wine is correlated with better nutrition in terms of type of fat (olive oil and other vegetable oils) and amount of fish, vegetables and fruits (high), animal protein and dairy food (low). Another possibility is that wine may be drunk in a healthier fashion than other alcoholic beverages. The traditional consumption of wine with meals may favourably influence post-prandial hyperlipidaemia. More indirect evidence is the decreasing consumption of wine and the stable CHD in France from 1961 to 1986 (Bellizzi et al. 1994).

The French Paradox and Longevity

It was tempting to use the term French paradox again after seeing the evolution of life expectancy in France compared to other European countries (Report from the Commission on the State of Health in the European Community 1996).

This increase in life expectancy is mainly due to the longevity figures for women. Women demonstrate a very low rate of cardiovcascular mortality and they drink very moderate quantities of wine and alcohol, avoiding the alcohol-related leading causes of mortality for men. They generally have better nutrition, especially in vegetables and cooked vegetables, which are the main contributors of carotenoids.

But nutrition cannot be the only explanation. The example of Sweden illustrates that other factors are involved. Looking at the evolution of cardiovascular disease incidence and mortality over the years of follow-up in the Monica study, the decrease in incidence rates of cardiovascular disease in the Northern part of France (urban community of Lille) compared to the rates in Toulouse was not accompanied by a similar decrease in mortality, even after controlling for access and type of health care. This finding is in line with the work of Marmot (1998), who showed that socio-economic considerations were important determinants of resistance to diseases and to their fatal evolution. He introduced the concept of "vulnerability" that results from complex interactions.

Physical environmental factors such as climate and especially insolation can play a role. Day-to-day variation in atmospheric pollutants has been shown to accelerate the fatal evolution of cardiovascular diseases. Therefore environmental and socio-economic factors have to be taken into consideration in addition to individual factors like nutrition and physical exercise.

Thus there is a wide range of determinants to explore, starting at the population level, with socio-economic characteristics and environmental factors (climate and pollution), to food pattern, which appear to be partly cultural and partly individual, to strictly individual factors, like the level of physical exercise, and last but not least genetics.

Genetic susceptibility to cardiovascular diseases and cancer can be investigated with molecular biology technics. Genetic polymorphism of apolipoproteins plays a role in cardiovascular disease incidence and polymorphism of phase I and II enzymes determines susceptibility to several types of cancer, like lung, colon-rectum and breast cancers.

This review of determinants of the main causes of death indicates the level of complexity of the factors involved in chronic degenerative diseases and, indirectly by extension, in longevity. It implies that there is no unique weapon in this struggle against death but a global attitude over life, within the context of given social conditions and genetic traits.

References

Artaud-Wild SM, Connor WE, Secton G (1993) Differences in coronary mortality can be explained by differences in cholesterol and saturated fat intakes in 40 countries but not in France and Finland. A paradox. Circulation 88:2771–2779

Bellizzi MC, Franklin MF, Duthie GG, James WPT (1994) Vitamin E and coronary heart disease: the European paradox. Eur J Clin Nutr 48:822–831

Corpet DE, Gerber M (1997) Alimentation méditerranéenne et Santé. I-caractéristiques. Maladies cardio-vasculaires et autres affections. Méd Nut 4:129–142

Criqui MH, Ringel BL (1994) Does diet or alcohol explain the French paradox? Lancet 344:1719–1723

Diaz MN, Frei B, Vita JA, Keaney JF (1997) Antioxidants and atherosclerotic heart disease. New Engl J Med 337:408–416

Ducimetiere P (1995) Le paradoxe français: mythe ou realite? Cah Nutr Diet 30:78–81

Ducimetiere P, Richard JL (1992) Dietary lipids and coronary heart disease: is there a french paradox? Nutr Metab Cardiovasc Dis 2:195–201

Duncan BB, Chambless LE, Schmidt MI, Folsom AR, Szklo M, Crouse JR, Carpentier MA (1995) Association of the waist-to-hip ratio is different with wine than with Beer or hard liquor consomption. Am J Epidemiol 142:1034–1038

Flatt JP (1995) Use and storage of carbohydrate and fat. Am J Clin Nutr, 61:S952–S959

Franceschi S, Favero A, Decarli A, Negri E, Lavecchia C, Ferraromi M, Russo A, Salvani S, Amadori D, Conti E, Montella M, Giacosa A (1996) Intake of macronutrients and risk of breast cancer. Lancet 347:1351–1356

Gerber M (1996) Fiber and breast cancer: another piece of the puzzle – but still an incomplete picture. J Natl Cancer Inst 88:857-858

Gerber M, Corpet D (1997) Alimentation méditeranéenne et Santé. II-Cancers. Méd Nut 4:143–154

Gerber M, Corpet D, Bougnoux Ph (1996) Equilibre énergétique et cancer, In: Riboli E, Decloitre F, Collet-Ribbing C (eds) Alimentation et cancer: Evaluation des données scientiofiques. Tec-Doc, Lavoisier, Paris, pp 255–280

Gjonça A, Bobak M (1997) Albanian paradox, another example of the protective effect of Mediterranean lifestyle? Lancet 350:1815–1817

Hertog MGL, Feskens EJM, Hollman PCH, Katan MB, Kromhout D (1993) Dietary antioxidants flavonoids and the risk of coronary heart disease: the Zutphen elderly study. Lancet 342:1007-1011

Kant AK, Schatzkin A, Harris T, Ziegler RG, Block G (1993) Dietary diversity and subsequent mortality in the first national health and examination survey epidemiologic follow-up study. Am J Clin Nutr 57:434–440

Knekt P, Jarvinen R, Seppanen R, Heliovaara M, Teppo L, Pukkala E, Aromaa A (1997) Dietary flavonoids and risk of lung cancer and other malignant neoplasms. Am J Epidemiol 146:223–230

Kushi LH, Lenart EB, Willett WC (1995) Health implications of Mediterranean diets in light of contemporary knowledge. 1. Plant foods and dairy products. 2. Meats, wine, fats, and oils. Am J Clin Nutr 61:S1407–S1427

Lissner L, Bengtsson C, Bjorkelund C, Wedel H (1996) Physical activity levels and changes in relation to longetivity. Am J Epidemiol 143:54–62

Marmot MG (1998) Improvement of social environment to improve health. Lancet 351:57–60

Møller H, Mellemgaard A, Lindvig K, Olsen JH (1994) Obesity and cancer risk: a Danish record-linkage study. Eur J Cancer 30A:344–350

Nube M, Kok FJ, Vandenbroucke JP, van der Heide-Wessel C, van der Heide-Wessel M (1987) Scoring of prudent dietary habits and its relation to 25-year survival. J Am Diet Assoc 87:171–175

Ortega RM, Requejo AM, Andres P, Lopez-Sobaler AM, Quintas ME, Rebondo MR, Navia B, Rivas T (1997) Dietary intake and cognitive function in a group of elderly people. Am J Clin Nutr 66:803–809

Perrig WJ, Perrig P, Stahelin HB (1997) The realtion between antioxidants and memory performance in the old and very old. J Am Geriatr Soc 45:718–724

Renaud S, de Lorgeril M (1992) Wine, alcohol, platelets and the French paradox for coronary disease. Lancet 339:1523–1526

Report from the Commission on the State of Health in the European Community, ECSE-EC-EAEC, Brussels. Luxembourg 1996

Serra-Majem L, Ribas L, Tresserras R, Ngo J, Salleras L (1995) How could changes in diet explain changes in coronary heart disease mortality in Spain? The Spanish paradox. Am J Clin Nutr 61S:1351S-1359S

Stoll BA (1994) Breast cancer: the obesity connection. Br J Cancer 69:799–801

WHO Monica Project (1994) Myocardial infarction and coronary deaths in the World Health Organization MONICA Project. Circulation 90:583–612

Willet WC (1997) Weight loss in the elderly: cause or effect of poor health? Am J Clin Nutr 66:737-738

Yu S, Derr J, Etherton TD, Kris-Etherton PM (1995) Plasma-cholesterol-predictive equations demonstrate that stearic acid is neutral and monounsaturated fatty acids are hypocholesterolemic. Am J Clin Nutr 61:1129–1139

Calorie Restriction: A Potent Mechanistic Solution to the Oxygen Paradox

B. P. Yu,[1] D. Y. Lee,[1] E. H. Hwang,[1, 2] and B. O. Lim[3]

Abstract

Although the oxidative stress theory of aging has gained popularity among many present-day gerontologists, the premise from which this hypothesis derives its basis is paradoxical because the same oxygen that supports life also threatens survival and causes aging. Until recently, no single experimental paradigm could offer satisfactory mechanistic explanations for this apparent self-contradiction to life. Recent investigations using the life-extending calorie restriction (CR) paradigm to investigate the modulation of free radical-induced oxidative stress, have produced sufficient data to support the notion that CR's anti-aging effect may come from its ability to tightly regulate the oxidative status of an organism. The result is the maintenance of cellular homeostasis, a hallmark of CR's action in the extension of life span. For example, recent findings on mitochondrial function and membrane structure indicate that, in an effort to guard against oxidative stress, membrane lipids synthesize with lower amounts of peroxidizable fatty acids. Mounting evidence shows membranes isolated from CR rats are much more stable and have a higher tolerance and stronger resistance to oxidative insult. These remarkable findings have been incorporated into the new "membrane peroxidation cycle" concept. The intervention of this cycle appears to be an evolutionary process that the CR rats have adapted as a strategy to protect the membrane in an oxidative environment.

Introduction

There is little doubt that aging is the most complex phenomenon seen in the biological systems of living organisms (Yu 1996). The intensified research of the last two decades has uncovered many interesting clues about the underlying aging processes of these systems, although many of the findings and conclusions resulting from such research have presented apparent paradoxes. For example, various

---

[1] Department of Physiology, The University of Texas Health Science Center, 7703 Floyd Curl Drive, San Antonio, TX 78284-7756, USA.
[2] On leave of absence from Wonkwang University, Iksan, Korea.
[3] On leave of absence from Kon Kuk University, Choongju, Korea.

J.-M. Robine et al. (Eds.)
Research and Perspectives in Longevity
The Paradoxes of Longevity
© Springer-Verlag Berlin Heidelberg New York 1999

experiments show life span extensions but with accompanying increases in morbidity or incidence of disease, or an extended life span only through reduced calorie intake, or the benefits of physical exercise with an increased oxygen consumption, which leads to increased oxidative stress.

One of the most significant breakthroughs in gaining mechanistic insights into such paradoxical phenomena is the calorie restriction (CR) paradigm. Reputed for its effectiveness, reproducibility, and diversity in modulating a broad spectrum of aging processes and disease pathogenesis, CR is currently the most highly regarded nutritional probe used by gerontologists in aging studies. The uniqueness of the CR paradigm makes it the most dependable and consistent probe to resolve the apparent oxygen paradoxes existing in aging phenomena.

CR as a Probe into the Aging Process

Before describing how the CR paradigm provides mechanistic insights into these apparent oxygen paradoxes, it is best to first describe how it became such a widely used probe in aging studies. Historically, the use of CR as a nutritional intervention in the aging process began with the work of Clive M. McCay, who was interested in establishing a long-suspected causal interrelation between an organism's rate of growth and its life span, i.e., aging (see review by Yu 1996). He accomplished this by testing what we now call the "growth retardation theory of aging," which claims that an organism's life span is inversely related to its growth rate. The reason that this theory became so prominent in the field of gerontology was due to the support of two other notions. The first notion is based on the interrelation of life span and metabolic rate, namely, that a slowing of the metabolic rate retards the aging process, thereby extending life span. The second notion implies that less "wear and tear" on bodily tissue slows the deterioration of biological systems. Until recently, each of these notions remained controversial due to the lack of systematic tests required for their experimental substantiation. However, as reliable evidence continues to accumulate, the validity of these simplistic notions is seriously called into question. More recent experiments using CR in rats initiated after sexual maturity show substantial life extensions – almost as good as life-long restriction – thereby negating the "growth retardation" theory of aging. In addition, convincing data from various experiments are now countering the "metabolic rate" theory by showing that CR and ad libitum (AL) fed rats have about the same metabolic rates.

CR as a Modulator of Oxidative Stress

More than any other theory of aging, the oxidative stress theory of aging, which encompasses all major theories of aging including those associated with mutation, DNA damage, glycation, and lipid peroxidation, offers the best in-depth molecular explanation for the processes responsible for most age-related deterioration, including pathological processes.

Over the past several years, free radical research has proven CR to be an effective modulator of life-shortening, free radical-induced cellular damage. This remarkable finding has provided investigators with a valuable tool to explore the mechanisms underlying the oxygen paradox. Our laboratory proposed that CR's ability to prolong the life span was dependent on its efficacy in regulating free radical metabolism (Yu 1996). Thus, the CR paradigm has become the most suitable tool of choice to resolve the many paradoxes observed in aging processes.

One outcome is exemplary of the studies that investigate the interrelation between an organism's metabolic rate and oxidative status. In the past, many gerontologists accepted without hard supporting data that metabolic rate, usually determined by the amount of O_2 consumed by an organism, is directly, inversely proportional to free radical generation. However, there is good reason to believe that such a simplistic relation is not supported by experimental evidence (Brierly et al. 1997; Forman and Azzi 1997). It should be noted, in fact, that the metabolic rate and the amount of oxygen consumed by CR animals are similar to those of AL fed animals (McCarter et al. 1997). The generation of reactive oxygen species in metabolically active tissue is expected to be nearly equal in both animals. This prospect raises important, interesting questions: 1) is the oxidative damage parallel in both CR and AL animals, and 2) what gives CR the ability to reduce oxidative status and extend life span? Recent research using the CR paradigm to investigate free radical metabolism has produced several important clues to resolve this paradox. CR has been shown to enhance an animal's ability to attenuate levels of potentially harmful reactive free radicals in various tissues (Yu and Yang 1996; Kristal and Yu 1998). This ability is evident in its effect on several aspects of free radical-related activities, including free radical generation, antioxidant-defense system activity (Yu 1994), and membrane (Choi et al. 1995; Kim et al. 1996) and DNA protection against free radical attack (Chunoj et al. 1992; Pieri 1997; Kang et al. 1998).

The maintenance of the membrane is especially important as its structural integrity is essential to proper cellular homeostasis (Zs-Nagy 1994). Recent studies offer substantial evidence that basic cellular membrane structures at all levels undergo oxidative alterations that elicit functional deficits (Yu 1996). Documented results show age-dependent deterioration in cellular homeostatic functions, such as many receptor-related functions, mitochondrial respiration, intracellular Ca^{2+} regulation, and signal transduction, all membrane-dependent activities (Hansford et al. 1997).

Thus, it is important to realize that CR's age-retarding abilities ameliorate age-related membrane deterioration, which no other putative intervention has ever shown, except for CR. Such effects should yield overall beneficial actions to preserve the integrity of the homeostatic condition. Therefore, it seems prudent that the focus of CR investigations should be on the cellular acitivities affected by free radical-induced membrane damage.

The Intervention of the Membrane Peroxidation Cycle by CR

The diverse effects of CR on the modulation of free radical-related processes are summarized in Table 1. As an outstanding membrane modifier, CR's ability to ward-off age-related membrane deterioration is the most suitable mechanistic explanation for the oxygen paradox. Among the most obvious modifications by CR are compositional changes related to membrane lipid composition, specifically, age-related membrane fatty acid composition (Laganiere and Yu 1993; Pieri 1997). This is an intriguing phenomenon, because until recently, it was unheard of for reduced calorie intake to alter membrane composition, although various dietary sources are known to change membrane composition. Even more intriguing is the way membrane compositional changes fend-off oxidative insult by suppressing the rise of polyunsaturation, which is compensated by increased 18:2 fatty acid. Evidence shows that, during aging, the membrane fatty acid profile tends to increase toward peroxidizable polyunsaturated acids, such as 22:4 and 22:5 (Devasagayam 1986; Laganiere and Yu 1993). Changes in the fatty acid profile can be taken as a compensatory mechanism for age-related membrane rigidity. However, the consequence of this compensatory increase in polyunsaturated fatty acids is an even higher state of peroxidizability, leaving the membrane even more susceptible to oxidative attack with exacerbated membrane rigidity (Pieri 1997). This paradoxical, vicious cycle is termed the "membrane peroxidation cycle" (MPC; Fig. 1). CR seems to modulate the fatty acid profile as a possible adaptive strategy to tolerate age-related oxidative damage, thereby preventing membrane deterioration (Pamplona et al. 1996).

An interesting action by CR is shown in its ability to intervene in the MPC by producing less highly peroxidizable acids, with an accompanying increase of linoleic acid (18:2) at the site of the cycle. In other words, the significance of an increase in 18:2 is that it is seemingly an adaptive action by the organism to properly maintain membrane fluidity without the risk of increased peroxidizability – an efficient, smart strategy to resolve the oxidative paradox. This strategy seems to develop in an evolutionary manner as an adaptive measure to fight oxi-

Table 1. Modulation of oxidative stress by dietary restriction

1. Generation of Reactive Species
   ◆ Superoxide
   ◆ H_2O_2
   ◆ Hydroxyl
   ◆ MDA
   ◆ 4-Hydroxynonenal
2. Lipid Peroxidation
3. Defense Systems
   ◆ Superoxide dismutase
   ◆ Catalase, peroxidase
   ◆ Glutathione
4. Iron Accumulation
5. Age-related Membrane Rigidity

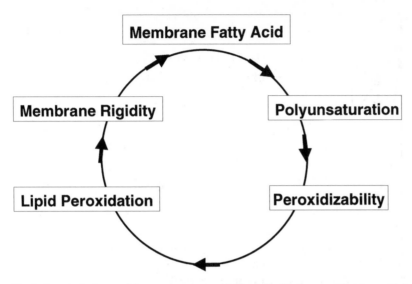

Fig. 1. Proposed scheme of the membrane peroxidation cycle. The increased lipid peroxidation due to age-related compositional changes in polyunsaturated fatty acids causes membrane rigidity. To maintain and compensate membrane fluidity, more polyunsaturated fatty acids are synthesized, causing the membrane to become more vulnerable to peroxidation. CR intervenes in this vicious cycle by maintaining membrane lipid composition with less peroxidizable fatty acids

dative damage, as shown in works by Barja's group (Pamplona et al. 1996). These investigators have shown differences in the life span of rats, pigeons, and humans through comparison studies of the degree of unsaturated fatty acid contents among these species. Their findings show that the extent of polyunsaturation (i.e., peroxidizability) inversely correlates with longevity (i.e., the higher the unsaturation, the shorter the life span), as was seen in short-lived rats compared with humans. Leading the way to the resolution of another paradox of aging, the species comparison shows that pigeons live eight to nine times longer than rats, despite having higher metabolic rates, which leads to the conclusion that the pigeons' longevity may be primarily attributed to increased resistance to lipid peroxidation due to lower polyunsaturated fatty acid levels. The CR paradigm seems to mimic an adaptive, evolutionary strategy for the survival of the organism when it is under oxidative stress.

Because membrane integrity is an essential requirement of cellular homeostasis, it seems that maintaining membrane integrity should be an organism's priority for survival, even in the case of limited calorie availability, as with CR. This survival strategy by an organism falls well within Kirkwood's general idea of the disposable soma theory, which proposes that an organism prioritizes energy utilization in an effort to maintain longevity of the species, which is necessary for survival (Kirkwood et al. 1997). Certainly, without properly maintained, essential cellular membrane integrity, survival is not possible (Zs-Nagy 1994; Yu 1996; Pieri 1997).

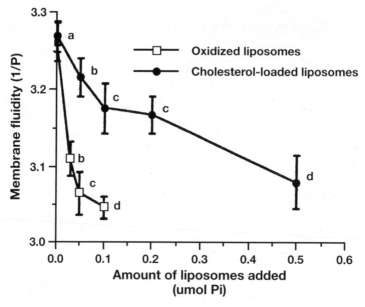

Fig. 2. Sensitivity of membrane fluidity to lipid peroxidation (Choi et al. 1995); □ oxidized-liposomes; ● cholesterol-loaded liposomes; a–d denote $p < 0.05$

   Observations made in our laboratory during the past few years show substantial age effects in the mitochondrial and microsomal membranes. We found further evidence to support CR's preventive action by documenting that age-related membrane rigidity is due to an extreme sensitivity to membrane lipid peroxidation (Fig. 2) and is not likely caused by increased membrane cholesterol. Contradicting the traditional view of age-related membrane rigidity, our studies show that the membranes of CR rats remain fluid even when the cholesterol/phospholipid ratio increases with age (Yu et al. 1992; Choi et al. 1995).

The Oxygen Paradox: Physical Exercise and CR

The eradication of infections disease, improved sanitation, personal hygiene, and the elimination of malnutrition have all contributed to increased life span. Yet, at the same time, modern conveniences have increased morbidity as populations have adopted sedentary lifestyles due to reduced amounts of physical acitvity. Our current sedentary lifestyle is considered a major underlying risk factor for disability in the elderly. There is little doubt that well-maintained physical activity is the best way to reduce the incidence of cardiovascular disease, diabetes, obesity, and other adult-onset disabilities. Rat experimentation clearly shows that exercise extends life span (Holloszy et al. 1985). Yet its metabolic demands require high oxygen consumption, which, in turn, causes possible oxidative damage – yet

Survival Curve

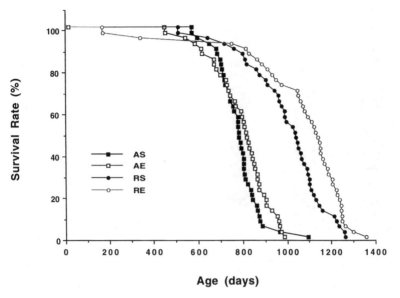

Fig. 3. Survival curve for the effect of exercise. AS, ad libitum fed, sedentary; AE, ad libitum fed, exercising; RS, CR, sedentary; RE, CR, exercising

another oxygen paradox. As one might expect, the production of reactive oxygen species in mitochondria increases during exercise. This phenomenon of the oxygen paradox has been observed in the increased lipid peroxidation (Ji and Leichtweis 1997) and DNA damage (Hartmann et al. 1995) detected in exercising subjects. However, it is important to note that, under proper conditions, this oxidative damage was shown to be substantially attenuated by the counteraction of the anti-oxidative defense systems, which are stimulated by exercise-induced oxidative stress. Thus, defense mechanisms play a key role in resolving the exercise-induced oxygen paradox.

Coupled with physical exercise, the CR paradigm provides another interesting way to explain the apparent oxygen paradox. A recent study (McCarter et al. 1997) reported data showing that CR animals that exercise have an additionally extended mean life span compared to their non-exercising CR counterparts (RE group in Fig. 3). How could this be possible if exercise promotes oxidative damage? The answer lies in CR's unique ability to withstand oxidative challenge. As the data show (Fig. 4), when mitochondria were challenged with the potent oxidant, butyl hydroperoxide, the mitochondria permeability of the CR rats was protected. Another interesting anti-oxidative action of CR is its ability to defend against the generation of damaging reactive oxygen species (ROS), which is expected to increase with exercise but is actually suppressed by CR (Fig. 5). Interestingly, the synergistic effect of the combined intervention of CR and exercise is

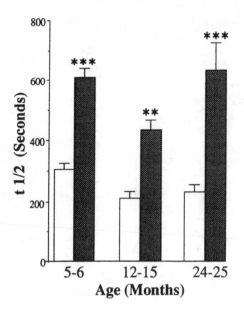

Fig. 4. Resistance to tert-butyl hydroperoxide challenge in mitochondria isolated from CR rats. The induction time for permeability transition was much prolonged compared to ad libitum fed controls. This shows CR ability to maintain a more stabilized membrane structure through increased resistance to oxidative stress. □ ad libitum fed controls; ■ CR rats
Diet-based statistical comparison: **, $p<0,05$; ***, $p<0,001$

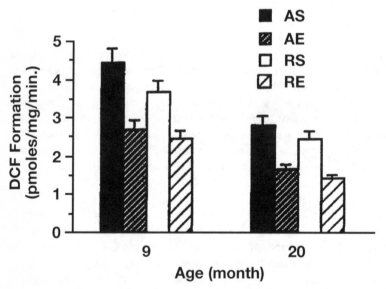

Fig. 5. Suppression of microsomal production of reactive oxygen species by CR. AS, ad libitum fed, sedentary; AE, ad libitum fed, exercising; RS, CR, sedentary; RE, CR, exercising; DCF = 2'-,7'-dichlorodihydrofluorescin

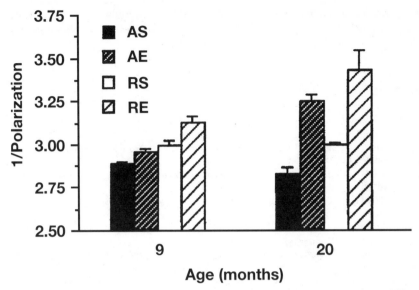

Fig. 6. Enhanced membrane fluidity by exercise. AS, ad libitum fed, sedentary; AE, ad libitum fed, exercising; RS, CR, sedentary; RE, CR, exercising

exemplified by the preservation of membrane fluidity (Fig. 6). Putting it all together, the evidence shows that exercising CR rats, despite having increased mitochondrial ROS production, have stronger mechanisms to defend against oxidative stress than non-exercising CR rats. The mechanisms for such a remarkable resistance to oxidative challenge are likely to come from the concerted effort of enhanced anti-oxidative defense systems (Yu 1996) and the suppression of peroxidizability of membrane fatty acids, as indicated in the intervention in the membrane peroxidation cycle by CR.

Summary

Theories and concepts of aging inundate the field of gerontology. Significant is the emergence of the free radical-based, oxidative theory of aging, which encompasses many existing theories. Theories relative to glycation, mutation, DNA damage, and nitric oxide could all fall under the oxidative stress theory. It is intriguing to know that this most versatile theory is fully supported by the life-extending effects of CR, as evidenced in the cellular events relating to the modulation of membrane composition and the antioxidant defenses essential to the maintenance of cellular homeostatis. In this presentation, "the membrane peroxidation cycle," in light of the effects brought about by CR, was discussed to highlight an adaptive membrane-stabilizing strategy for longevity, much like the evolutionary processes observed in long-lived species. The CR paradigm deserves recognition not only for its protective effect in maintaining cellular homeostasis by attenuating oxidative stress, but also for its ability to modulate the "membrane peroxidation cycle," thereby in providing us with a mechanistic explanation for some of the apparent paradoxes that exist in aging processes.

References

Brierley EJ, Johnson MA, James OFW, Turnbull DM (1997) Mitochondrial involvement in the ageing process: Facts and controversies. Mol Cell Biochem 174:325–328

Choi MC, Jackson C, Yu BP (1995) Lipid peroxidation contributes to age-related membrane rigidity. Free Rad Biol Med 18:977–984

Chung MH, Kasai H, Nishimura S, Yu BP (1992) Protection of DNA damage by dietary restriction. Free Rad Biol Med 12:523–525

Devasagayam TPA (1986) Low level of lipid peroxidation in newborn rats: Possible factors for resistance in hepatic micosomes. FEBS Lett 199:203–307

Forman HJ, Azzi A (1997) On the virtual existence of superoxide anions in mitochondria: Thoughts regarding its role in pathophysiology. FASEB J 1:374–375

Hansford RG, Houge BA, Mildaziene V (1997) Dependence of H_2O_2 formation by rat heart mitochondria on substrate availability on donor age. J Bioenerg Biomemb 29:89–95

Holloszy JO, Smith EK, Vining M, Adam S (1985) Effect of voluntary exercise on longevity of rats. J Appl Physiol 59:826–831

Hartmann A, Nieb AM, Grünert-Fuch M, Poch B, Speit G (1995) Vitamin E prevents exercise-induced DNA damage. Mutation Res 346:195–202

Ji LL, Leichtweis S (1997) Exercise and oxidative stress: Source of free radicals and their impact on antioxidant systems. AGE 20:91–106

Kang CM, Kristal BS, Yu BP (1998) Age-related mitochondrial DNA deletions: Effect of dietary restriction. Free Rad Biol Med 24:148–154

Kim JD, McCarter RJM, Yu BP (1996) Influence of age, exercise, and dietary restriction on oxidative stress in rats. Aging Clin Exp Res 8:123–129

Kirkwood TBL (1997) Is there a biological limit to the human life span? In: Robine LM, Vaupel JW, Jeune B, Allard M (eds.) Longevity: To the limits and beyond. Springer-Verlag, Berlin pp. 69–76

Kristal BS, Yu BP (1998) Resistance to oxidant-mediated inhibition of mitochondrial transcription. AGE, in press

Laganiere S, Yu BP (1993) Modulation of membrane phospholipid fatty acid composition by age and food restriction. Gerontology 39:7–18

McCarter RJM, Shimokawa I, Ikeno Y, Higami Y, Hubbard GB, Yu BP, McMahan CA (1997) Physical activity as a factor in the action of dietary restriction on aging: Effects in Fischer 344 rats. Aging Clin Exp Res 9:73–79

Pamplona R, Prat J, Cadena S, Rojas C, Pérez-Camp R, Lopez M, Barja TG (1966) Low fatty acid unsaturation protects against lipid peroxidation in liver mitochondria from long-lived species: The pigeon and human case. Mech Ageing Dev 86:53–66

Pieri C (1997) Membrane properties and lipid peroxidation in food restricted animals. AGE 20:71–79

Yu BP (1994) Cellular defenses against damage from reactive oxygen species. Physiol Rev 74:139–162

Yu BP (1996) Aging and oxidative stress: Modulation by dietary restriction. Free Rad Biol Med 21:651–668

Yu BP, Suescun EA, Yang SY (1992) Effect of age-related lipid peroxidation on membrane fluidity and phospholipase A_2: Modulation by dietary restriction. Mech Ageing Dev 65:17–33

Yu BP, Yang R (1996) Critical evaluation of the free radical theory of aging: A proposal for the oxidative stress hypothesis. Ann NY Acad Sci 786:1–11

Zs-Nagy I (1994) The membrane hypothesis of aging. CRC Press. Boca Raton, FL

Linguistic Ability in Early Life and Longevity: Findings from the Nun Study

D. A. Snowdon[1,2], L. H. Greiner[1], S. J. Kemper[3], N. Nanayakkara[1], and J. A. Mortimer[4]

Abstract

Findings from the Nun Study indicate that low linguistic ability in early life has a strong relationship to poor cognitive function and dementia in late life and to the number of Alzheimer's disease lesions in the brain. In the present analyses, we investigated the relationship between linguistic ability in early life and all cause mortality in late life in a subset of 180 participants in the Nun Study. Two measures of linguistic ability in early life – idea (proposition) density and grammatical complexity – were derived from autobiographies written by the participants when they were 18 to 32 years old. An average of 58 years later, when these participants were 75 to 93 years old, all cause mortality rates were determined. Of the two linguistic measures, idea density in early life had the strongest and most consistent relationship to the rate of all cause mortality in late life. A one-unit decrease in idea density in early life (i. e., one fewer idea expressed per 10 words in a sentence) was associated with a 49 % increase in the mortality rate (95 % CI = 17–89; p-value = 0.001). This finding did not appear to be due to confounding by birth year, education attained at the time when the autobiography was written, or age during the mortality suveillance period. Standard life table analyses indicated that the median age at death for 75-year-olds was 81.7 years for those with low idea density in early life and 88.5 years for those with high idea density in early life. Low linguistic ability in early life may reflect suboptimal cognitive and neurological development that may increase susceptibility to aging-related declines and disease processes, resulting in a higher mortality rate late in life. Overall, low linguistic ability and its correlates in early life may place potent limits on the longevity of individuals.

[1] Sanders-Brown Center on Aging.
[2] Department of Preventive Medicine, College of Medicine, University of Kentucky, 101 Sanders Brown Bldg, Lexington, KY 40536-0230, USA.
[3] Psychology Department, University of Kansas, Lawrence, KS, USA.
[4] Institute on Aging, University of South Florida, Tampa, FL, USA.

J.-M. Robine et al. (Eds.)
Research and Perspectives in Longevity
The Paradoxes of Longevity
© Springer-Verlag Berlin Heidelberg New York 1999

Background

Low attained education is associated with poor health and function in older adults (Snowdon et al. 1989 a, b; Pincus et al. 1987; Folsom et al. 1989) and a higher risk of Alzheimer's disease and dementia (Zhang et al. 1990; Dartigues et al. 1991; Fratiglioni et al. 1991; Stern et al. 1994; Mortimer and Graves 1993). Individuals with low education may be more likely to develop dementia and other diseases because of lifestyle differences associated with education, such as nutrition, alcohol consumption, and occupational exposures. An alternate explanation is that low education reflects suboptimal cognitive and neurological development in early life, and that suboptimal brain development may increase susceptibility to aging-related declines and disease processes late in life.

Neurocognitive development in early life may be marked by other variables besides years of formal education. We have proposed that linguistic ability in early life reflects important aspects of cognitive ability, neurocognitive development, and neurologic reserve (Snowdon et al. 1996). Findings from the Nun Study indicate that low linguistic ability in early life has a strong relationship in late life to poor cognitive function, risk of dementia, and the number of Alzheimer's disease lesions in the brain (Snowdon et al. 1996). In the present study, we investigated the association between linguistic ability in early life and all cause mortality in late life.

Women included in the present analysis were participants in the Nun Study, a longitudinal study of aging and Alzheimer's disease (Snowdon et al. 1996, 1997; Snowdon 1997). While it may be difficult to generalize from this unique population of Catholic sisters, many factors that confound most epidemiologic studies have been minimized or eliminated. Participants in our study had the same reproductive and marital histories; had similar social activities and support; did not smoke, or drink excessive amounts of alcoholic beverages; had similar occupations, income, and socioeconomic status; lived in similar houses; ate food prepared in similar kitchens; and had comparable access to preventive, nursing, and other medical care services.

Methods

Study Population

Participants in the Nun Study are members of the School Sisters of Notre Dame religious congregation and live in communities in the Midwestern, Eastern, and Southern United States. The design of this longitudinal study has been described in detail elsewhere (Snowdon et al. 1996, 1997 b; Snowdon 1997) and will only be described briefly here. At the first exam in 1991–1993, the 678 participants were 75 to 102 years old (mean = 83). Cognitive and physical function were assessed annually and all participants agreed to brain donation at death. As described below, the present analysis was conducted on a subset of 180 participants who had handwritten autobiographies from early life.

Linguistic Measures

In September 1930, the leader of the School Sisters of Notre Dame in North America requested that each sister" ... write a short sketch of her own life. This account should not contain more than two to three hundred words and should be written on a single sheet of paper ... include the place of birth, parentage, interesting and edifying events of one's childhood, schools attended, influences that led to the convent, religious life, and its outstanding events ... ."

Handwritten autobiographies were found in the convent archives for 180 US-born sisters who took their religious vows during 1931 to 1943. All of these autobiographies were written within two years before the sisters took their vows and formally joined the religious congregation. All of the autobiographies were written by sisters who entered either the Milwaukee, Wisconsin or Baltimore, Maryland convents. While sisters in other convents may have written autobiographies during the same time period, handwritten autobiographies for such sisters did not exist in the convent archives. Thus, the sample used in the present analysis was made up of the 180 US-born Milwaukee and Baltimore sisters with handwritten autobiographies from early life. These 180 sisters represent 83 % of the 218 US-born participants in the Nun Study who took their vows in these convents during 1931 to 1943.

Two indicators of linguistic ability were derived from each autobiography: idea density (Kintsch and Keenan 1973; Turner and Greene 1997) and grammatical complexity (Cheung and Kemper 1992). Prior studies suggest that idea density is associated with educational level, vocabulary, and general knowledge, whereas grammatical complexity is associated with working memory, performance on speeded tasks, and writing skill (Kemper et al. 1989, 1990, 1992; Cheung and Kemper 1992; Kemper 1990; Lyons et al. 1993).

In the present analysis, the mean idea density and grammatical complexity scores of each sentence were computed for the last 10 sentences of each autobiography. Idea density was defined as the average number of ideas expressed per 10 words. Ideas corresponded to elementary propositions, typically a verb, adjective, adverb, or prepositional phrase. Complex propositions that stated or inferred causal, temporal, or other relationships between ideas were also counted. Grammatical complexity was computed using the Developmental Level metric originally developed by Rosenberg and Abbeduto (1987) and modified by Cheung and Kemper (1992). The Developmental Level metric classifies sentences according to eight levels of grammatical complexity, ranging from zero (simple one-clause sentences) to seven (complex sentences with multiple forms of embedding and subordination).

Without the linguistic coders' knowledge of the age or cognitive function of each sister during late life, each autobiography was scored for idea density and grammatical complexity. The inter-coder correlation was 0.88 for idea density and 0.93 for grammatical complexity for the Milwaukee participants, and 0.83 for idea density and 0.96 for grammatical complexity for the Baltimore participants.

The following excerpts from autobiographies illustrate the method used to compute idea density (ID) and grammatical complexity (GC):

"I was born in Eau Claure, Wis., on May 24, 1913 and was baptized in St. James Church. (ID=3.9,GC=0)

The good example given to me by my teachers and the true religious spirit that they showed did much in directing my steps to Notre Dame. (ID=4.2,GC=7)

In nineteen hundred thirty-two I was admitted into the "hallowed precincts" of the Novitiate which was a happy, holy time. (ID=8.0,GC=3)

Now I am wandering about in "Dove's Lane" waiting, yet only three more weeks, to follow in the footprints of my Spouse, bound to Him by the Holy Vows of Poverty, Chastity, and Obedience. (ID=9.1,GC=7)."

The ideas expressed in the first sentence were 1) I was born, 2) born in Eau Claire, Wis., 3) born on May 24, 1913, 4) I was baptized, 5) was baptized in church, 6) was baptized in St. James Church, and 7) I was born ... and was baptized. There were 18 words or utterances in that sentence. The idea density for that sentence was 3.9 (i.e., 7 ideas divided by 18 words and multiplied by 10 resulting in 3.9 ideas per 10 words).

Statistical Methods

All deaths among the participants were recorded for the period between November 13, 1991, and March 1, 1998 (i.e., the mortality surveillance period started at the first exam). Cox proportional hazards regression was used to model the relationship between linguistic ability in early life and risk of death in late life. Using methods described by Korn et al. (1997), the time scale for the regression was age at entry into the mortality surveillance period (i.e., age at the first exam) and age at exit from the mortality surveillance period (i.e., age at death or, if alive, age on March 1, 1998). Use of age as the time scale allows for a more direct comparison of the risk of death during the mortality surveillance period among participants of like ages than does the use of years observed in the study as the time scale (Korn et al. 1997). Furthermore, by stratifying the regression model based on birth year, the use of age as the time scale allows for the resulting model to adjust for age, birth year, and calender year during the mortality surveillance period (since birth year plus age equals calender year during the mortality surveillance period).

Stratified Cox proportional hazards regression models were used to adjust for selected variables: 1) age during the mortality surveillance period (i.e., using age as the time interval for the regression model, as described above), 2) birth year cohort (i.e., four strata based on the quartile distribution of birth year), 3) convent (i.e., two strata based on whether the participants were from the Milwaukee or Baltimore convents), 4) education at the time the autobiography was written (i.e., three strata based on whether the participant had less than a high school diploma, had only a high school diploma, or had a bachelor's or master's degree), 5) the presence of dementia at the beginning of the mortality surveillance period (i.e., two strata based on whether or not the participant met our dementia criteria; Snowdon et al. 1997), and 6) the Mini-Mental State Exam score at the beginning of the mortality surveillance period (i.e., this measure of global cognitive function was included as a covariate in the regression model).

The regression models were used to derive the relative risk of death, which refers to the ratio of mortality rates (or, more exactly, the ratio of hazards functions from the regression model). In addition, standard life table methods were used to apply age-specific all cause mortality rates (deaths per person-years observed) to a hypothetical group of 75-year-olds in order to estimate the cumulative percentages surviving to selected ages and the median age at death.

Results

Descriptive Data

All 180 participants took their vows and joined the religious congregation during 1931 to 1943 at either the Milwaukee, Wisconsin convent (n = 101) or the Baltimore, Maryland convent (n = 79). All participants were white, of European heritage, and born in the United States. Each participant wrote an autobiography some time between the ages of 18 and 32 (mean = 22). At that time, 18 % had less than a high school education, 76 % had earned a high school diploma, and 6 % had earned a bachelor's or master's degree. An average of 58 years after writing the autobiographies, when the participants were 75 to 91 years old (mean = 80), they began to participate in the Nun Study. By that time, 91 % of them had earned bachelor's degrees.

Milwaukee (M) participants were similar to Baltimore (B) participants on the mean age when they wrote the autobiographies (M = 22, B = 22), the percent who eventually earned a bachelor's degree or higher (M = 92 %, B = 90 %), and the mean age at which they began to participate in the Nun Study (M = 80, B = 80). Milwaukee and Baltimore participants did differ, however, on the percentage of participants who had less than a high school education when they wrote the autobiographies (M = 10 %, B = 29 %; p < 0.001).

There also were differences between the two convents in the distributions of the two linguistic measures derived from the autobiographies written in early life. The Milwaukee participants had a higher mean idea density score (M = 6.9, B = 5.0; p = 0.0001), whereas the Baltimore participants had a higher mean grammatical complexity score (M = 2.8, B = 4.4; p < 0.0001). The differences between the convents in the distributions of the two linguistic measures were also apparent later in life. At the third annual exam in the Nun Study, sisters were asked to write a short autobiography. Of the 180 participants assessed at the first exam, 139 survived to the third exam and 127 were cognitively and physically able to write autobiographies. The late life autobiographies were similar to the early life autobiographies, i.e., those from Milwaukee had a higher mean idea density score (M = 5.5, B = 3.6; p = 0.0001), whereas those from Baltimore had a higher mean grammatical complexity score (M = 2.4, B = 2.9; p = 0.006). Overall, Milwaukee participants appear to have placed greater emphasis on the expression of ideas, thoughts, and emotions, whereas Baltimore participants appear to have placed greater emphasis on sentence structure.

Mortality Data

During the mortality surveillance period of November 13, 1991, to March 1, 1998, the 180 participants ranged in age from 75 to 93 years, and 58 (32%) of them died (M = 34%, B = 30%). Table 1 shows findings for the relationship between the linguistic measures from early life (ages 18 to 32) and the risk of all cause mortality in late life (ages 75 to 93). In these analyses, each linguistic measure from early life was treated as a continuous variable. Grammatical complexity in early life had a weak and inconsistent relationship with the risk of mortality and was therefore not considered in subsequent analyses. In contrast, idea density in early life had a statistically significant negative association with the risk of mortality within each convent and in both convents combined. Among all partici-

Table 1. Linguistic ability in early life and all cause mortality in late life among 180 participants in the Nun Study

Linguistic measures from early life	Variables adjusted in the analyses besides age and birth year[a]	Convent	Relative risk of death associated with one unit decrease in linguistic measure (95% CI)		P-value
Idea density		Milwaukee	1.36	(1.03–1.79)	0.03
		Baltimore	1.90	(1.22–2.98)	0.005
		Both	1.49	(1.17–1.89)	0.001
	Education	Milwaukee	1.47	(1.08–1.98)	0.01
		Baltimore	1.81	(1.14–2.88)	0.01
		Both	1.56	(1.21–2.02)	0.001
	Education and grammatical complexity	Milwaukee	1.45	(1.07–1.97)	0.02
		Baltimore	1.81	(1.05–3.13)	0.03
		Both	1.53	(1.17–1.99)	0.002
Grammatical complexity		Milwaukee	1.23	(0.81–1.85)	0.33
		Baltimore	1.63	(0.95–2.79)	0.08
		Both	1.37	(0.97–1.92)	0.07
	Education	Milwaukee	1.23	(0.81–1.87)	0.34
		Baltimore	1.35	(0.78–2.33)	0.28
		Both	1.27	(0.91–1.78)	0.16
	Education and idea density	Milwaukee	1.14	(0.77–1.69)	0.53
		Baltimore	1.00	(0.55–1.81)	0.99
		Both	1.12	(0.81–1.54)	0.50

[a] As described in the methods, age was adjusted by using age as the time scale in the regression, whereas the other variables were adjusted by stratification. Stratification by convent also was done in the analyses for both convents combined. The linguistic measures were adjusted by their inclusion as covariates in the regression model.

pants, a one unit decrease in idea density in early life (i.e., one fewer idea expressed per 10 words in a sentence) was associated with a 1.49 relative risk of death, after adjusting for birth year and age during the mortality surveillance period (95 % CI = 1.17–1.89; p-value = 0.001). That is, each one unit decrease in idea density was associated with a 49 % increase in the mortality rate (or more exactly, a 49 % increase in the hazard function derived from the regression model).

The inverse relationship between idea density and mortality was present after adjusting for education (Table 1). Furthermore, to strictly control for education, additional age-and birth year-adjusted analysis was done on the subset of 137 participants who had only a high school diploma when they wrote their early life autobiographies. For these participants, a one unit decrease in idea density in early life was associated with a 1.48 relative risk of death (95 % CI = 1.13–1.95; p-value = 0.005).

Other age- and birth year-adjusted findings for all 180 participants indicated that the relationship between idea density in early life and risk of mortality in late life was stronger during younger ages. A one unit decrease in idea density in early life was associated with a 2.61 relative risk of death during ages 75 to 79; a 1.55 relative risk during ages 80 to 84; and a 1.12 relative risk during ages 85 to 89 (95 % CI = 1.10–6.23, p-value = 0.03; 1.16–2.08, 0.003; and 0.70–1.81, 0.63, respectively).

Additional findings suggest that the relationship between idea density in early life and risk of mortality in late life is due to the associations between idea density, cognitive function, and mortality. Among all 180 participants, a one unit decrease in idea density in early life was associated with a 1.49 relative risk of death after adjusting for age and birth year; a 1.18 relative risk after additional adjustment for the presence of dementia at the start of the mortality surveillance period; and a 0.96 relative risk after further adjustment for the participants' Mini-Mental State Exam scores at the start of the mortality surveillance period (95 % CI = 1.17–1.89, p-value = 0.001; 0.90–1.56, 0.24; and 0.70–1.33, 0.82, respectively).

Table 2 shows additional findings on the relationship between idea density in early life and risk of mortality in late life. Because of the previously described differences in the distribution of idea density between convents, idea density was categorized based on its distribution by quartiles within each convent. Within each convent, and in both convents combined, an excess risk of death appeared to be largely confined to the bottom quartile of the distribution of idea density in early life. For the remaining analyses, low idea density refers to the bottom quartile of scores and high idea density to the top three quartiles within each convent. Overall in both convents combined, the age- and birth year-adjusted relative risk of death in the low idea density group was 2.65 (95 % CI = 1.50–4.67; p-value = 0.001) when compared to the high idea density group (Table 2).

Table 3 shows the results of age-specific analyses on the relationship between idea density in early life and the risk of mortality and likelihood of survival during late life. Using standard life table methods, the age-specific mortality rates in

Table 2. Idea density in early life and all cause mortality in late life among 180 participants in the Nun Study

Convent	Idea density in early life (quartile)[a]	Participants dead/at-risk	Deaths per 100 person-years	Relative risk of death (95 %) CI[b]		P-value
Baltimore	(1)	11/20	15	2.92	(0.95–8.96)	0.06
	(2)	5/21	5	0.89	(0.25–3.10)	0.85
	(3)	3/15	4	0.72	(0.17–3.04)	0.65
	(4)	5/23	4	1.00		
	Low (1)	11/20	15	3.33	(1.36–8.15)	0.01
	High (2,3,4)	13/59	4	1.00		
Milwaukee	(1)	13/25	14	2.99	(1.05–8.54)	0.04
	(2)	6/25	5	1.02	(0.29–3.63)	0.98
	(3)	10/28	8	1.90	(0.64–5.59)	0.25
	(4)	5/23	4	1.00		
	Low (1)	13/25	14	2.27	(1.08–4.74)	0.03
	High (2,3,4)	21/76	6	1.00		
Both	(1)	24/45	14	2.92	(1.36–6.25)	0.01
	(2)	11/46	5	0.96	(0.39–2.34)	0.93
	(3)	13/43	6	1.36	(0.59–3.12)	0.47
	(4)	10/46	4	1.00		
	Low (1)	24/45	14	2.65	(1.50–4.67)	0.001
	High (2,3,4)	34/135	5	1.00		

[a] For the Milwaukee participants the quartile (Q) distribution of idea density was: Q1 = 3.9–5.8, Q2 = 5.9–7.1, Q3 = 7.2–7.8, and Q4 = 7.9–9.3. For the Baltimore participants it was: Q1 = 2.3–4.5, Q2 = 4.6–5.3, Q3 = 5.4–5.5 and Q4 = 5.6–6.9

[b] As described in the methods, age was adjusted by using age as the time scale in the regression, whereas birth year cohort was adjusted by stratification. Stratification by convent also was done in the analyses for both convents combined

Table 3. Idea density in early life and age-specific all cause mortality and survival in late life among 180 participants in the Nun Study

Idea density in early life	Age interval	Participants dead/at-risk	Deaths per 100 person-years	Cumulative percent[a] survived to	
				Start of interval	End of interval
Low	75–79	2/17	8	100	68
	80–84	17/34	18	68	28
	85–89	4/17	10	28	17
High	75–79	3/80	2	100	92
	80–84	20/126	6	92	69
	85–89	11/51	10	69	43

[a] As described in the Methods, the findings were derived using standard life table techniques. While the findings above were similar within each convent, findings are only presented for both convents combined in order to increase the sample sizes in the youngest and oldest age intervals

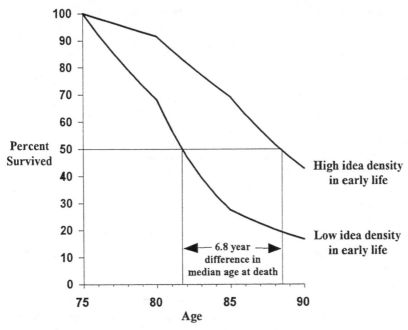

Fig. 1. Idea density in early life and the cumulative percent survival to different ages in late life among 180 participants in the Nun Study

Table 3 were applied to a hypothetical group of 100 75-year-olds in order to calculate the cumulative percentages surviving to specific ages (Table 3 and Fig. 1). These analyses indicated that 17 % of 75-year-olds with low idea density in early life would survive to age 90, compared to 43 % of those with high idea density in early life. Furthermore, the median age at death for 75-year-olds was 81.7 years for those with low idea density and 88.5 years for those with high idea density in early life, resulting in a 6.8-year difference in median age at death.

Comments

Our findings support a strong inverse relationship between linguistic ability in early life and the risk of mortality in late life. Low linguistic ability, as indicated by low idea density demonstrated in autobiographies written at an average age of 22 years, was significantly associated with a high risk of all cause mortality 58 years later. Our findings did not appear to be due to confounding by birth year, education at the time the autobiography was written, or age during the mortality surveillance period. As in our previous findings on cognitive function and Alzheimer's disease (Snowdon et al. 1996), idea density in early life had a stronger and more consistent association with all cause mortality than did grammatical complexity.

We suspect that the relationship of low linguistic ability in early life to the risk of all cause mortality in late life has more to do with the linguistic and cognitive abilities of the participants in early life than to lifestyle and environmental risk factors present during mid and late adult life. Participants in the Nun Study had the same reproductive and marital histories; had similar social activities and support; did not smoke, or drink excessive amounts of alcohol; had similar occupations, income, and socioeconomic status; lived in similar houses and ate food prepared in similar kitchens; and had comparable access to preventive and medical care services. This high level of comparability and the absence of several confounding factors largely offset the reduced generalizability of the findings from this special population. The relative homogeneity of the sisters' adult lifestyles and environments suggests that sisters with low linguistic ability in early life brought risk factors with them when they joined the religious congregation at an early age.

Low linguistic ability in early life may reflect suboptimal neurological and cognitive development that might increase susceptibility to aging-related declines and disease processes late in life. Our prior research indicates that those with low linguistic ability in early life have a greater risk of clinically and neuropathologically confirmed Alzheimer's disease, and a greater number of Alzheimer's disease lesions in the brain, than those with high linguistic ability (Snowdon et al. 1996). In the present study, the relationship between linguistic ability in early life and all cause mortality in late life was eliminated when we controlled for impaired cognitive function in late life in the analyses. An increased rate of development of Alzheimer's disease lesions in the brain may explain the high risk of death in late life among those with low linguistic ability. Overall, low linguistic ability and its correlates in early life may place potent limits on the longevity of individuals.

Acknowledgments

This study would not have been possible without the spirited support of the members, leaders, and health care providers of the School Sisters of Notre Dame religious congregation. The following were especially helpful in the present study: Sisters Sarita Genin, Rita Mae Gruenke, Margaret Karas, Louis Marie Koesters, Alice Lechnir, Marlene Manney, Marie Kevin Mueller, Marjorie Myers, Francita Orcholski, and Gabriel Mary Spaeth; and Huaichen Liu MD, William Markesbery MD, Ela Patel, Jeanne Ray, and Cecil Runyons. Gari-Anne Patzwald MS provided invaluable editorial assistance. This study was funded by grants R01AG09862 (Dr. Snowdon), K04AG00553 (Dr. Snowdon), and 5P50AG05144 (Dr. Markesbery) from the National Institute on Aging, and grants from the Abercrombie Foundation and the Kleberg Foundation. More information about the Nun Study may be obtained by visiting our web page: http://www.coa.uky.edu/nunnet

References

Cheung H, Kemper S (1992) Competing complexity metrics and adults' production of complex sentences. Appl Psycholing 13:53–76

Dartigues JF, Gagnon M, Michel P, Letenneur L, Commenges D, Barberger-Gateau P, Auriacombe S, Rigal B, Bedry R, Alpérovitch A, Orgogozo JM, Henry P, Loiseau P, Salamon R (1991) Le programme de recherche Paquid sur l'épidémiologie de la démence. Méthodes et résultats initiaux. Rev Neurol (Paris) 147: 225–230

Folsom AR, Prineas RJ, Kaye SA, Soler JT (1989) Body fat distribution and self-reported prevalence of hypertension, heart attack, and other heart disease in older women. Int J Epidemiol 18:361–367

Fratiglioni L, Grut M, Forsell Y, Viitanen M, Grafström M, Holmén K, Ericsson K, Bäckman L, Ahlbom A, Winblad B (1991) Prevalence of Alzheimer's disease and other dementias in an elderly urban population: relationship with age, sex, and education. Neurology 41:1886–1892

Kemper S (1990) Adults' diaries: changes made to written narratives across the life span. Discourse Processes 13:207–223

Kemper S, Kynette D, Rash S, O'Brien K, Sprott R (1989) Life-span changes to adults' language: effects of memory and genre. Appl Psycholing 10:49–66

Kemper S, Rash S, Kynette D, Norman S (1990) Telling stories: the structure of adults' narratives. Eur J Cogn Psych 2:205–228

Kemper S, Kynette D, Norman S (1992) Age differences in spoken language. In: West RL, Sinnott JD (eds) Everyday memory and aging. Springer-Verlag, New York NY, pp 138–152

Kintsch W, Keenan J (1973) Reading rate and retention as a function of the number of propositions in the base structure of sentences. Cogn Psych 5:257–274

Korn EL, Graubard BI, Midthune D (1997) Time-to-event analysis of longitudinal follow-up of a survey: choice of the time-scale. Am J Epidemiol 145:72–80

Lyons K, Kemper S, LaBarge E, Ferraro F, Balota D, Storandt M (1993) Language and Alzheimer's disease: a reduction in syntactic complexity. Aging Cogn 50:81–86

Mortimer JA, Graves AB (1993) Education and other socioeconomic determinants of dementia and Alzheimer's disease. Neurology 43:S39–S44

Pincus T, Callahan LF, Burkhauser RV (1987) Most chronic diseases are reported more frequently by individuals with fewer than 12 years of formal education in the age 18–64 United States population. J Chron Dis 40:865–874

Rosenberg S, Abbeduto L (1987) Indicators of linguistic competence in the peer group conversational behavior of mildly retarded adults. Appl Psycholing 8:19–32

Snowdon DA (1997) Aging and Alzheimer's disease: lessons from the Nun Study. Gerontologist 37:150–156

Snowdon DA, Ostwald SK, Kane RL (1989a) Education, survival, and independence in elderly Catholic sisters, 1936–1988. Am J Epidemiol 130:999–1012

Snowdon DA, Ostwald SK, Kane RL, Keenan NL (1989b) Years of life with good and poor mental and physical function in the elderly. J Clin Epidemiol 42:1055–1066

Snowdon DA, Kemper SJ, Mortimer JA, Greiner LH, Wekstein DR, Markesbery WR (1996) Linguistic ability in early life and cognitive function and Alzheimer's disease in late life: findings from the Nun Study. JAMA 275:528–532

Snowdon DA, Greiner LH, Mortimer JA, Riley KP, Greiner PA, Markesbery WR (1997) Brain infarction and the clinical expression of Alzheimer's disease: the Nun Study. JAMA 277:813–817

Stern Y, Gurland B, Tatemichi TK, Tang MX, Wilder D, Mayeux R (1994) Influence of education and occupation on the incidence of Alzheimer's disease. JAMA 271:1004–1010

Turner A, Greene E (1977) The construction and use of a propositional text base. University of Colorado Psychology Department, Boulder CO.

Zhang M, Katzman R, Salmon DP, Jin H, Cai G, Wang Z, Qu G, Grant I, Yu E, Levy P, Klauber MR, Liu WT (1990) The prevalence of dementia and Alzheimer's disease in Shanghai, China: impact of age, gender, and education. Ann Neurol 27:428–437

Personality and Longevity: Paradoxes

H. S. FRIEDMAN[1]

There is a long history of research and theory arguing that certain patterns of psychological responding are damaging to or promoting of physical health – that is, that certain personalities are disease-prone or self-healing (Friedman 1990, 1991). It is often assumed that people who are sociable, optimistic, undemanding, and easygoing are prone to health and longevity, but the research designs have been weak, and contradictory examples are common.

During the past eight years, these issues of personality and longevity have been examined using the longest-running and most comprehensive relevant data set (Friedman et al. 1995a). The participants were 1,528 bright Californians who were recruited as boys and girls by Lewis Terman in 1922 (at an average age of 11 years), and who have been studied intensively ever since. More than half of them are now dead, and we have gathered their death certificates and coded their dates and causes of death. These life-span data provide a unique opportunity to address intriguing questions about the role of personality in longevity using a longitudinal, prospective design. Statistical survival analyses (hazard regressions) were employed to predict longevity from psychosocial and behavioral factors.

A number of paradoxes have emerged. Why is sociability (and popularity) not predictive of longevity, despite the known association between social support and health? Why do cheerful and optimistic children grow up to be at higher risk of premature mortality than their more sober counterparts? What is the personality trait that is most strongly associated with longevity?

Background

Some of the roots of this work evolved in Paris over 100 years ago with the ideas of Claude Bernard, the great 19th-century French physiologist. Bernard emphasized the "mileur interne" – the internal environment – the idea that all living things must maintain a constant or balanced internal environment. This idea of equilibrium and homeostasis was further developed by Hans Selye (1976) with his notion of a General Adaptation Syndrome to stress, and by Walter Cannon (1932), who wrote about the Wisdom of the Body – the never-ending fight for stabilization.

[1] University of California, Riverside, CA 92521 USA.

J.-M. Robine et al. (Eds.)
Research and Perspectives in Longevity
The Paradoxes of Longevity
© Springer-Verlag Berlin Heidelberg New York 1999

These scientists further understood, however, that the body has to remain in equilibrium not only inside but also outside. That is, the person has to be in balance with the environment to remain healthy. Certain people fit best with (match) the environment. More than that, we now know that people create and help seek out their environments (Caspi and Bem 1990). The situations we find ourselves in are not totally random. So, much attention needs to be focused on the psychology of the individual – that is, on the qualities of personality that keep one healthy or make one more prone to disease and early death.

In psychosomatic medicine, assorted theories argue that certain patterns of psychological responding are damaging to or promoting of physical health. It is often assumed that people who are sociable, upbeat, undemanding, and easygoing are prone to health and longevity; tenseness, struggle, too much work, seriousness, and introversion are often thought to be unhealthy. In the 1940's, Franz Alexander, a leading proponent of psychosomatic medicine, described the cases of two middle-aged women with breast cancer. Two years after mastectomy, Ginny was dying but Celia was back at her job with new responsibilities. Alexander (1950) could not find a biological explanation for the different outcomes – the tumors were similar. So, he looked for personality differences. He found that Ginny bragged about how brave she was, and repeatedly asserted that she was going to get well, but she seemed unable to face her disease or her feelings about losing her breast. Celia, on the other hand, was neither excessively optimistic nor full of despair. She admitted that losing a breast was hard and tried to find out how she could adjust. Celia recovered but Ginny died. Are such psychological factors of balance really so relevant to health? Relatedly, are some active, hurried, workaholic people healthy (both physically and mentally), despite the fact that they seem to be "Type A" (Friedman and Booth-Kewley, 1987)? How can this be?

The Terman Data

Groucho Marx reportedly said, "Anyone can get old. All you have to do is live long enough." However, such reasoning is not enough for science; we need to collect good data.

The participants in our studies were 1,528 bright Californians who were recruited as boys and girls by Lewis Terman in 1922 (at an average age of 11 years), and who have been intensively studied ever since. More than half of them are now dead. These life-span data provide a unique opportunity to address intriguing questions about the role of personality in longevity, using a longitudinal, prospective design. Statistical survival analyses (hazard regressions) were employed to predict longevity from personality and behavioral factors.

The Terman Life Cycle study (formerly called the Genetic Studies of Genius; Terman and Oden 1947) aimed at securing a reasonably random sample of bright California children, and so most public schools in the San Francisco and Los Angeles areas were searched for students, nominated by their teachers and tested by Terman to have an IQ of at least 135. There were 856 boys and 672 girls in the study; they have been followed at five- to ten-year intervals ever since.

To make this archive suitable to address longevity questions, our project has gathered and coded death certificates, gathered and refined certain data about smoking, and developed many new indexes (of personality and health behavior) necessary for studying longevity and cause-of-death effects. In this remarkable study, only small percentages (less than 10 %) of the participants are unaccounted for. (Size varies somewhat with the subsample of each analysis.) We generally restrict our analyses to those who were of school age in 1922, who lived at least until 1930, and for whom there are not substantial missing data. Our childhood personality measures come from 1922 and our adult health behaviors, adult personality, and adult adjustment measures come from mid-life (usually 1950, but ranging from 1940–1960). This typically results in a sample size of between 1,100 and 1,300. Analyses by Terman's researchers as well as our own comparisons indicate that those lost from the study do not differ systematically.

The sample is not representative of the U.S. population as a whole (for example, it contains less than 1 % Asian-, African-, or Native-Americans). Results, especially effect sizes, are not necessarily generalizable to populations different on health-relevant dimensions. However, there is the usual variation in personality, and many relations between personality and longevity should not be much different in different populations. On the positive side, certain counfounds common to other psychosocial health studies are not likely here. The participants could understand medical advice and prescription, had adequate nutrition, and had access to medical care. The participants had regular contact with Stanford University. Explanations of poor health involving poverty, ignorance, or discrimination are generally not applicable to this sample, and so the sample is valuable for focusing on personality variables. Also, the participants were successful in public school, at least to the extent that they made it through teachers' nominations and Terman's tough screening for intellectual talent; this is important to keep in mind since it helps rule out certain competing explanations for longevity. Finally, the longitudinal design of the present study points out the importance of not focusing too heavily on short-term coping with stress to the exclusion of lifelong habits and patterns.

Findings

We initially examined all items collected by Terman in 1922 that seemed relevant to personality. In 1922, one of the subject's parents (usually the mother, or both parents together) and the subject's teacher were asked to rate the subject on 25 trait dimensions chosen to measure intellectual, volitional, moral, emotional, aesthetic, physical, and social functioning. Each of these 25 traits was rated on a 13-point scale, according to the degree to which the child appeared to possess each trait. The scales used are remarkably modern in their appearance (Friedman et al. 1993).

We constructed six personality dimensions from childhood and used them to predict longevity and cause of death through 1986, using survival analyses (see Friedman et al. 1993, 1995a, b). We then used adult measures (from 1940 and 1950). We used both Cox proportional hazards and Gompertz regressions; they yielded the same results. Does personality predict premature mortality decades later?

Conscientiousness/Social dependability

"Conscientiousness/social dependability" was measured by the four items of prudence, conscientiousness, freedom from vanity/egotism, and truthfulness. It is reasonable to expect that parents and teachers have a good idea of whether an 11-year-old child is conscientious, prudent, and so on. This corresponds roughly to the "Big Five" dimension of Conscientiousness. However, some notions of conscientiousness include a "need for order", a notion not captured in our dimension; rather, our conscientiousness scale may have also captured some elements (such as honesty) of what is sometimes termed "Agreeableness" (Costa et al. 1991). The Cronbach's alpha for this scale was .76, indicating good reliability.

The most striking finding in these and follow-up analyses is that this childhood social dependability or conscientiousness is predictive of longevity. Conscientious children, especially boys, live significantly longer throughout the lifespan. They are about 30 % less likely to die in any given year. This finding is also confirmed on analyses of these participants as adults.

Survival analyses (n = 1,215) on cause of death suggest that the protective effect of conscientiousness is partially but not primarily due to a reduction in the risk of injury: Although there is some tendency for the unconscientious to be more likely to die a violent death (homicide, suicide, accident), conscientiousness is also protective against early death due to cardiovascular disease and cancer.

Sociability/Extroversion

Despite the known health correlates of social support, this study has found no evidence that the personality trait of sociability or other elements of extroversion are strongly related to longevity in this sample. This is paradoxical, given that one assumes that sociability will bring social support. For example, childhood ratings on such variables as "popularity" and "preference for playing with other people" did not predict longevity. Does an extroverted child who grows up to be a fast-talking salesman or a glad-handing politician really lead a more balanced life?

To further explore the lifelong effects of sociability, we followed up on Terman's (1954) study of scientists. Terman had found that the participants who grew up to be scientists (broadly construed) were much less sociable early in life than the non-scientists. (Only male scientists were studied by Terman.) In fact, Terman considered the differences in sociability to be quite remarkable. Using the Stanford archives, we re-created Terman's groups (n = 288 and 326), and compared their longevity through 1991. However, our survival analyses found that the scientists did not die sooner. In fact, the scientists tended to live longer (relative hazard = 1.26, p<0.09; Friedman et al. 1994). Paradoxically, these bright, well-educated but introverted boys grew up to lead stable, interesting lives.

Neuroticism and Adult Adjustment

It is known that special groups such as the clinically depressed or criminals are more likely to face early death (such as from suicide or homicide), but the relation between psychological adjustment and premature mortality is little studied in long-term, prospective population research. Emotional instability, depression, and hostility are found to be correlated with poor health in various other studies, but what are results in this current sample? Results are mixed. On the childhood measures, there is some hint that neuroticism may be unhealthy, although it is proving challenging to create valid measures of neuroticism since it is desirable to take various elements of the lifelong reaction patterns into account. For example, for males, permanency of mood (as rated in childhood) tended to be associated with increased longevity. Here again, stability predicts longevity.

What about in adulthood? In 1950, the Terman participants were asked about tendencies toward nervousness, anxiety, or nervous breakdown; there also had been personal conferences with participants and with family members. Based on this and on previous related information in the files dating back a decade, Terman's team then categorized each on a three-point scale of mental difficulty: satisfactory adjustment, some maladjustment, or serious maladjustment. (Almost one-third experienced at least some mental difficulty by this stage.) Survival analyses show that for males, mental difficulty as of 1950 significantly predicted mortality risk through 1991, in the expected direction. Similar results were found on a measure we constructed of poor psychological adjustment as self-reported in 1950 on six 11-point scales such as "moodiness" (Martin et al. 1995).

On cause of death, there are no dramatic differences as a function of psychological adjustment. A general survival analysis model testing for differences among causes of death (cardiovascular disease, cancer, injury, other disease) shows no significant difference. That is, poorly adjusted people are more likely to die from all causes. There is some indication that poorly adjusted participants are especially more likely to die from injury (including suicide), as would be expected. However, since so few people die from injury in this sample, such differences cannot (and do not) account for the main effect of adjustment on longevity.

Cheerfulness (Optimism and Sense of Humor)

It may be helpful to be optimistic when one is facing trauma or the necessity of recovering from disease, but this may not necessarily be generally health-protective across the life-span. Examining childhood cheerfulness – rated as optimism and a sense of humor – this study found, contrary to expectation, that childhood cheerfulness is inversely related to longevity. Survival analyses showed that the cheerful children grew up to be adults who died sooner (about 22 % increased risk, p <0.01).

Puzzled, we have followed up on those Terman participants rated as cheerful in childhood. We found that they grew up to be more likely to smoke, drink, and take risks (all p's <0.05), although these habits do not fully explain their increased risk of premature mortality. Cheerfulness may be helpful when facing a stress such as surgery, but harmful if it leads one to be careless or carefree throughout one's life (Tennen and Affleck 1987; Weinstein 1984). Also, some cheerfulness may also be a cover-up for psychological pain. In other words, the health relevance of such traits as optimism needs to be more carefully conceptualized (cf. Wortman et al. 1992). This does not mean that the dour and depressed people are especially healthy; rather, it implies that excessive cheerfulness is not necessarily a sign of homeostasis, and in fact, may be a part of a more reckless life.

Health Behaviors

Can cigarette smoking and heavy use of alcohol (which often occur together) account for these personality differences in longevity? Using Terman's 1950 and 1960 surveys, we classified the participants as heavy drinkers, as moderate drinkers (seldom or never intoxicated), or as rarely (or never) taking a drink. (Alcohol use was quite stable across decades.) Since moderate drinking may be protective of heart disease, we also looked for U-shaped effects on mortality, but none were found. Information about smoking was poorly documented in the files, and so we collected as much smoking information as possible during 1991–1992. Unlike the other measures, there is some evidence of bias in this subsample. Those who died young seem more likely to have had very unhealthy behaviors, and also were less likely to have locatable families; the mediating effect of smoking may thus be underestimated due to missing data.

As expected, smoking and drinking each predicted premature mortality. Did they mediate the relations reported above? Conscientious children grew up to drink and smoke less, but cheerful kids grew up to drink and smoke more (all p's <0.05). However, conscientiousness remains a strong predictor of longevity in various survival analyses, controlling for smoking and drinking (decreased hazard of 20–30 %). Cheerfulness remains predictive when alcohol use is controlled, but the effects of Cheerfulness change when smoking is controlled; since the sample size drops by one-third, what this means is problematic. Females participants who faced the stress of parental divorce grew up to smoke more (p < 0.05) but not drink more (possibly due to Prohibition during adolescence), and this explains their increased risk.

Psychosocial factors might affect a whole host of health behaviors in addition to drinking and smoking – exercise patterns, diet, use of prophylactics, adherence to medication regimens, avoidance of environmental toxins, and more –

which, when put together, may explain most of the associations between psychology and longevity. Surprisingly, there is little prospective study of psychosocial predictors of unhealthy lifestyle patterns across long time periods and how they subsequently and consequently affect health, longevity, and cause of death. These matters are currently being investigated.

In sum, the data concerning unhealthy behavior are tantalizing but not definitive. Personal factors evident in childhood are predictive of smoking and excessive drinking in adulthood, and these unhealthy behaviors predict premature mortality in this sample. Yet these behaviors do not come close to fully accounting for the effects of childhood predictors on longevity. It may be the case that more reliable and more extensive measurement of health behaviors could demonstrate a major impact in explaining the psychosocial predictors of longevity, without resort to psychosomatic explanations involving stress. Given the documented associations of stress with both cardiovascular disease mechanisms and suppression of the immune system, however, it is likely that there are multiple pathways linking personality to longevity. A reasonable supposition is that personality has both direct (psychosomatic) and behaviorally-mediated effects on health, but ascertaining their relative importance is a difficult empirical question.

Conclusion

Mohandas K. Ghandi (also called Mahatma or "Great Soul") faced much work, stress, struggle, and hardship. Yet he was not sickly, even after spending over 2300 days in prison and enduring numerous self-imposed fasts. On the contrary, he had the personal strength and commitment to be one of the most influential leaders of the 20th century, and perhaps of all time. He pioneered nonviolent political resistance, instituted numerous social reforms, and won political freedom for India. He was assassinated in his 78th year. What defined Ghandi's life was a commitment to principle. As he aged, he grew more content with his life, but remained humble. He certainly was not blindly optimistic or happy-go-lucky. He loved people but was not a flirt. To understand his health, we need to see the whole way he led his life. This is sadly missing from many analyses of personality and longevity, which are too short or narrow.

The most sophisticated analyses of longevity increasingly recognize that research must proceed simultaneously on various complementary fronts. There are biological influences set in motion by genetic and prenatal endowments, and there are subsequent biological influences of infections, traumas, toxins, oxidation, nutrition, and so on throughout life. On the psychosocial and behavioral side, there are the stresses, coping styles, addictions, health behaviors, habits, and socio-cultural networks, which are often intertwined with the biological factors. The present paper focuses expertise on the Terman data set, which is exceptionally well-suited to analyze one particular piece of the larger puzzle – individual differences in personality as they unfold across the life-span, from childhood in the 1920's through old age in the 21st century. We see that paradoxes can be resolved if we examine the full story of an individual's characteristics and how that individual lives his or her life.

Overall, problems in psychosocial adjustment related to an egocentric impulsivity turn out to be a key general risk factor for all-cause mortality. The locus of health-relevant effects seems to be centered in such traits as impulsivity, egocentrism, toughmindedness, and undependability. Although common wisdom might argue that a selfish, self-indulgent, reckless lout may prosper by stepping on others, this does not seem to be the case. Nor do we find a triumph of the lazy, easygoing, pampered drop-out, nor of the eternal optimist. In terms of the rush towards death, the encouraging news is that the good, dependable, conscientious folks finish last.

References

Alexander F (1950) Psychosomatic medicine. New York, Norton

Cannon W (1932) The wisdom of the body. NY: Norton

Caspi A, Bem DJ (1990) Personality continuity and change across the life course. In: Pervin LA (ed) Handbook of personality: Theory and research. New York, Guilford Press, pp. 549–575

Costa PT, McCrae R, Dye DA (1991) Facet scales for agreeableness and conscientiousness: A revision of the NEO Personality Inventory. Personality Indiv Diff 12:887–898

Friedman HS (1990) Personality and disease. New York, Wiley & Sons

Friedman HS (1991) Self-healing personality: why some people achieve health and other succumb to illness. New York, Henry Holt

Friedman HS, Booth-Kewley S (1987) Personality, type A behavior, and coronary heart disease: The role of emotional expression. J Personality Soc Psychol 53:783–792

Friedman HS, Tucker J, Tomlinson-Keasey C, Schwartz J, Wingard D, Criqui MH (1993) Does childhood personality predict longevity? J Personality Soc Psychol 65:176–185

Friedman HS, Tucker JS, Martin LR, Tomlinson-Keasey C, Schwartz JE, Wingard DL, Criqui MH (1994) Do non-scientists really live longer? The Lancet 343:296

Friedman HS, Tucker JS, Schwartz JE, Tomlinson-Keasey C, Martin LR, Wingard DL, Criqui MH (1995a). Psychosocial and behavioral predictors of longevity: The aging and death of the "Termites." Am Psychol 50:69–78

Friedman HS, Tucker J, Schwartz JE, Martin LR, Tomlinson-Keasey C, Wingard D, Criqui M (1995b). Childhood coscientiousness and longevity: Health behaviors and cause of death. J Personality Soc Psychol 68:696–703

Martin LR, Friedman HS, Tucker JS, Schwartz JE, Criqui MH, Wingard DL, Tomlinson-Keasey C (1995). An archival prospective study of mental health and longevity. Health Psychol 14:381–387

Selye H (1976) The stress of life (rev. ed.). New York, McGraw-Hill

Tennen H, Affleck G (1987) The costs and benefits of optimistic explanations and dispositional optimism. J Personality 55:377–393

Terman LM (1954) Scientists and nonscientists in a group of 800 gifted men. Psychol Monographs 68:1–44

Terman LM, Oden MH (1947) Genetic studies of genius: The gifted child grows up. Vol. 4. Stanford, CA, Stanford University Press

Weinstein N (1984) Why it won't happen to me. Perceptions of risk factors and susceptibility. Health Psychol 3:431–457

Wortman CB, Sheedy C, Gluhoski V, Kessler RC (1992) Stress, coping, and health: Conceptual issues and directions for future research. In: Friedman HS (ed) Hostility, coping and health. American Psychological Assn, Washington, DC, pp 227–256

Dying Healthy or Living Longer: A Society's Choice[1]

J. Légaré[2] and Y. Carrière[3]

"Agir non en connaissance de cause, mais en connaissance des conséquences."
Druet, 1990

As the 21st Century nears, industrialized countries have reached very low levels of mortality and fertility. This phenomenon is characterised by demographers as the last stage of the demographic transition theory. These almost universal levels were reached, for the most part, thanks to technological advances that only a century ago were not imaginable. Although the development of new technologies raised great debates on the ethics of their indiscriminate application in the field of human reproduction, the same cannot be said for the secular drop in mortality. Further lowering mortality, or prolonging life, seems to be an unassailable objective, regardless of the methods used.

Furthermore, predicting the future of mortality has never been a perilous exercise for demographers, even though they often have been mistaken as life expectancy has always been longer than forecasted. Critics were not strict concerning this conservatism, a legacy of actuaries, since the consequences could only satisfy the populations that always dreamed of living longer, with death being linked to a certain fatality.

But is the battle against death acceptable at any cost? Significant progress in mortality reduction in industrialized countries automatically entails an increase in the aging process of the population. Thus, the spectre of our society's accelerated aging has frayed more than one decision maker, particularly those interested in social policies and more specifically those in the health sector.

While in the past it has been mainly the decrease in fertility that has influenced the aging of the population, the decrease in mortality has nevertheless played a role that cannot be ignored and that will only increase over time (Caselli and Vallin 1990). However, a reduction in mortality does not automatically imply a healthier society. We can ask ourselves the question whether or not it is more important to live one's old age in health or to prolong life needlessly.

The context of the evolution of scientific progress will force certain choices, conscious or unconscious, between living better and living longer. There are several issues at stake in this debate and the objective of this presentation is to define

[1] This article is a revised and updated translation of Légaré and Carrière, 1991.
[2] Department of Demography, University of Montreal, P. O. Box 6128 Succ. Centre Ville, Montreal, Quebec H3C3J7, Canada.
[3] Simon Fraser University, Vancouver, Canada.

J.-M. Robine et al. (Eds.)
Research and Perspectives in Longevity
The Paradoxes of Longevity
© Springer-Verlag Berlin Heidelberg New York 1999

the markers of possible choices and to make decision makers aware of the consequences of their choices. After a brief overview of the evolution of mortality and
morbidity as they have been measured in the past and predicted for the future,
we will support our position by showing the social and ethical implications of
prolonging life expectancy whatever the costs.

The Mortality and Morbidity Trends

The Recent Past

The recent trend of life expectancy shows a tendency towards a continuous rise,
both for men and for women. In industrialized countries, life expectancy has
gone from 60 years one-half century ago to 80 years now. The increase has been
quicker for women, who originally were already at an advantage over men. Such
an outcome has created a gap in life expectancy between sexes that has increased
progressively, sometimes reaching as much as 10 years.

The gains that were reached primarily in the younger age groups means that
more and more people are reaching the threshold of old age. However, for several
years now, the elderly have benefited from more and more gains on mortality,
allowing not only more of them to reach age 65 but also to live well beyond that
age (Table 1).

Table 1. Number of Survivors to Age 65 (I_{65}) per 100.000 Persons at Birth and Life Expectancy at age
65 (e_{65}), by sex, Canada, Birth Cohorts 1801–1941

Birth Cohort	Canada			
	I_{65}		e_{65}	
	Males	Females	Males	Females
1801	27,448	31,092	10.64	11.54
1811	28,560	32,708	10.72	11.62
1821	29,640	34,115	10.86	11.81
1831	30,769	35,552	11.08	12.09
1841	31,959	37,017	11.38	12.48
1851	33,529	38,793	12.10	13.09
1861	35,901	40,968	12.89	13.83
1871	40,401	44,734	13.24	14.57
1881	44,909	49,331	13.48	15.65
1891	47,131	53,035	13.62	17.19
1901	51,561	59,715	14.03	18.65
1911	57,716	66,910	14.70	20.09
1921	63,984	74,131	15.86	21.16
1931	68,362	78,219	17.22	22.20
1941	74,502	83,380	18.00	22.42

Source Bourbeau et al. 1997

Unfortunately, we have much less information about the evolution of the health status of populations, partially because health status is a more recent concern and the indicators are less reliable and more difficult to compare over time as well as from country to country.

Regardless of these limits, we can calculate a disability-free life expectancy, which is an indicator, not a measurement, of the health status of populations. To calculate such an indicator, the number of years lived in institutions or with permanent or temporary restrictions of activity must be subtracted from the total number of years lived. Thus, it becomes possible to evaluate, among other things, the quality of the life expectancy gains made in recent years.

A recent study (Robine et al. 1995) clearly indicates the complexity of the situation. Regardless of the limitations of comparisons in time and space, life expectancy without severe disability seems to evolve in a fashion parallel to life expectancy (Fig. 1), which would confirm Manton's theory of the "dynamic equilibrium" (Manton 1982).

However, all levels combined of disability-free life expectancy either stagnates or increases at a lesser rate than life expectancy (Fig. 2). A similar trend has recently been observed for the USA up to the 1990s (Crimmins et al. 1997). Most of the extra years of life achieved would be years of disability.

Upon examination of disability-free life expectancy at age 65, this phenomenon becomes even more apparent (Robine et al. 1995, p 14). Almost half of those years lived are, on average, years lived in poor health, and the gap observed between men and women for life expectancy almost disappears when we compare disability-free life expectancy. Such a statement has to be qualified, however, when more in-depth information is available (Cambois et al. 1997).

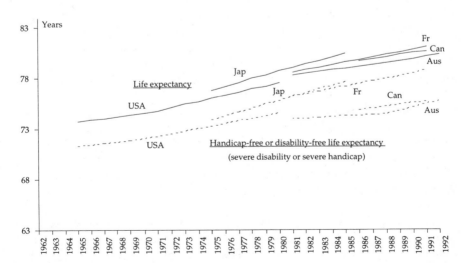

Fig. 1. Severe handicap-free or severe disability-free life expectancy, for females at birth. International comparison from 1965 to 1991. Source: Robine et al. 1995

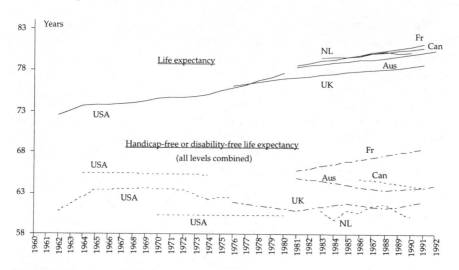

Fig. 2. Handicap-free or disability-free life expectancy, all levels combined, for females at birth. International comparison from 1965 to 1991. Source: Robine et al. 1995

These results allow us to qualify the immense progress made in the recent battle against mortality. Given present morbidity rates, a high life expectancy does not necessarily mean a better health status of the population.

Some Future Scenarios

We can also illustrate these secular mortality and morbidity trends by survival curves of which life expectancy is a summary indicator (Fig. 3). We can also plotted an optimal survival curve, almost rectangular, picturing our present knowledge when eliminating premature deaths (Duchene and Wunsch 1988).

Furthermore, the surface between the two curves – that of the survivors with all health status combined and that of the disability-free survivors – is directly proportionate to the years lived in poor health (Fig. 3a). The supplementary years recently gained push the survival curve to the right without the equivalent displacement on the disability-free curve. While there is a definite increase in the number of years lived, they are for the most part lived in poor health. This leaves us not too far from the optimal survival curve, in conformity with the situation where there are fewer and fewer premature deaths (Fig. 3b). Such a phenomenon is referred to by demographers and epidemiologists as the rectangularisation of the survival curve.

Fries, however, goes farther than this mortality compression. He suggests that in the near future we could also experience a morbidity compression. Therefore, both curves would reach more or less the optimal survival curve (Fig. 3b) and the number of years lived in poor health would be reduced to a minimum (Fries 1980).

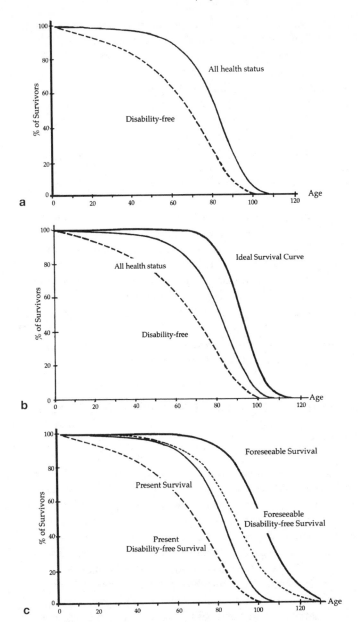

Fig. 3. Total life expectancy and disability-free life expectancy. A) Present situation: Total survival curve and disability-free survival curve. B) Ideal situation: Mortality and morbidity compression with only a single disability-free survival curve. C) Foreseeable situation: rectangularisation of the total survival curve without morbidity compression. Source: Légaré and Carrière 1991

This scenario does not foresee any further important progress in lengthening longevity, but does imply that the number of years of disability has been reduced as much as possible. We would live a little bit longer and we would die healthy ... of old age.

For some, however, substantially increasing life expectancy is an objective that could be attained in the near future (Walford 1983; Manton 1991), and recent progress in immunology foresees a slowing down of the aging process (Bodnar et al. 1998). In this scenario, not only is the mean age at death pushed beyond 100 years, but the age at which the disability process begins is also pushed proportionately (Fig. 3c). Here, we would live much longer, but we would die after having lived a certain number of years of disability, comparable to the present situation.

Whether future generations live the Fries scenario or the Manton scenario will not be simple fate. For some, these theories conflict. But we go further by asserting that, beyond the fact that these theories are pertinent and regardless of the needed progress in fighting factors related to youth death rates (car accidents, AIDS, etc.), the future of morbidity and mortality will reflect the allocation of resources to elderly health care and the weight given to geriatric research within bio-medical research as a whole. Regardless of the costs and the prestige associated with these choices, policy makers should take into account present day value systems. We must separate the good from the bad, or at least find a "lesser" bad. As a result, everything becomes a question of ethics or social justice.

Desirable Evolution from Life to Death and the Value System

Medicine and Health Care

The links between medicine and longevity raise many debates. We will look at the links between medicine and health care before trying to picture the future.

Since the turn of this century, medicine's contribution to the improvement of life expectancy has often been questioned (Kunitz 1987, 1991). Most of today's epidemiologists believe that medicine has historically had a relatively small impact on the improvement of life expectancy, yet this is not to say that the impact has been negligible (Kuntzmann 1997). More importance is given to such factors as hygiene, economic conditions, lifestyle, etc. (Wilkins and Adams 1983; Cribier 1997). These studies demonstrate that a more global approach towards illness is necessary. The state, in its role as health care manager, should favour a policy aimed at preventive medicine.

While the state is well aware of the benefits of preventive medicine, it is technology that receives a significant part of the funds allocated to the health system. There is much opposition to this situation. The main objections raised by opponents to massive investment into new technologies are primarily:

– that costs are too high and reduce the amount available for research and preventive medicine;

– that the efficiency of these techniques to improve the population's health status is questionable.

We are not trying to call into question all sophisticated technologies; rather, we are primarily discussing some technology and extraordinary care intended for the elderly. However, the use of these new technologies more often than not simply delays by a few days an inevitable death without providing the individual with any extra autonomy. The exorbitant costs of prolonging life without improving the health status of the patient create an increase in morbidity and social costs of illness. This situation can hardly be viewed as economically efficient. It these resources were used in a preventive manner, the mortality differences between socio-economic classes would no doubt be reduced and the life expectancy of less favoured groups would improve.

An analysis of the health care costs during the last year of life indicates that the imminence of death often goes hand in hand with high costs, without the health status, particularly the autonomy of the patient, necessarily improving (Fuch 1984; Roos et al. 1987; Felder and Meier 1996). These costs then limit the amounts available for other fields of medicine and welfare.

To fully understand the debate surrounding the use of technologies and sophisticated care to delay imminent death, one must remember that the death of a patient is considered a failure in the eyes of the medical community. If technology is successful in prolonging life, there is an increase in life expectancy. While there is effectively a quantitative improvement, the medical community interprets it as a success, a victory. Questioning such practices affects the basic principles of medicine.

Medicine and Longevity

Is it possible to imagine prolonging life in a significant manner? As seen earlier, more and more people are reaching the threshold of old age. They are also surviving longer on average, thus the important improvement in total life expectancy, even if throughout this entire period of progress, the maximum life span for humans has only slighthly increased (Thatcher, 1999). The result of this evolution is the more and more pronounced rectangularisation of the survival curve (Fig. 3).

Is it idealistic to believe that mortality will become a phenomenon that affects the population within such a short age interval that there will be systematic rectangularisation of the survival function?

While there are several different opinions on the subject (Schneider and Brody 1983; Myers and Manton 1984; Fries 1984), the debate does not take away from what is at stake. If rectangularisation does take place, then is it impossible to aim for morbidity compression (Schneider and Guralnick 1987; Wilkins 1987; Wilkins and Adams 1987)? Two conditions are necessary for this phenomenon to occur. Firstly, the present limit on life expectancy bounderies must be seen as societaly acceptable, and secondly, we must target to delay the onset of morbidity.

Fries believes this scenario to be eventually possible. However, it would be more realistic to imagine a partial morbidity compression. To achieve this, the average age at which permanent disabilities tend to occur must rise at a rate faster than that of life expectancy. Such an objective implies a certain vision of medicine. Research efforts must be geared towards prevention of those ailments that tend to bring about disability – blindness, deafness, arthritis, fractures, etc. Action on these ailments has little to do with mortality (Myers 1988) but has important consequences on the quality of life, especially after age 60 (Egidi and Frova 1997, p 310). Projecting medicine in such a way puts the biomedical research model into question. Accepting such an approach is equivalent to admitting defeat against unchangeable limits for human life or at least a postponement of a breakthrough. Is the medical community ready to accept such a position (Callahan 1990)? That would then mean questioning the use of non-curative sophisticated care aimed at the elderly, care that is extremely costly and usually only serves to prolong suffering.

The morbidity compression theory touches both moral and professional values that are difficult to call into question. In addition, the theory implies the re-allocation of funds already available to the health care system. Our societies should demonstrate their maturity and tackle this debate very soon.

Ethics and Health Care

The debate that surrounds sophisticated care for the elderly is too often linked to the present socio-economic context as well as to efficient allocation of our health care system's resources (Callahan 1987). Little consideration is taken for more humanitarian values.

Value of Life

Our societies recognize several rights of the patient, but not yet the right to die. What can an analysis of the ethics theory provide, that we may see the issues more clearly? According to John Rawls, the structure of an ethics theory is largely determined by the manner in which it defines and links notions of what is good and what is fair (Rawls 1971). If we define life as a "good," then we must define the quality of that life as "fair." An ethical theory of medicine would therefore make the link between life and the quality of life.

Reverend Jack Gallagher once stated the following concerns about health care: "The aim of health care is to preserve life and this goal seems to me to be primordial above all other considerations." Further on, he asks the following questions: "Should we be ready to spend whatever necessary in order to ensure the life and health of a person, or are there limits which should not be crossed? If there are limits, what are they?" (Gallagher 1987).

The value given to life per se surely must not be questioned. But isn't the boundary of these limits, for all practical purposes, the point at which the battle against death becomes a battle against life? While these limits cannot be expressed monetarily, they can be expressed in suffering or simply in respect for the human being. The boundary is determined by negotiating between the good and the fair, between life and the quality of life. By ignoring what is fair, we are condemning life to be interpreted as having a value without limits, to the detriment of human dignity.

Prolonging Life or Improving the Quality of Life

Equity is needed in allocating the resources within the health care system. In many countries, the system provides for universal health care. In other words, "to each according to his needs." Since health tends to deteriorate with age, this type of policy entails high costs in order to meet the needs of the elderly. The sophisticated technology used to keep the elderly alive only contributes to the growth of these costs. But does this technology respond to an actual need? If there is a need, then should there not be also a demand? (Barer et al. 1995) Would it not be more advantageous for society to opt for an improvement in the quality of life rather than expensively attempt to prolong life? This is especially true given that future gains in life expectancy, as small as they may be, could only be achieved through a large increase in public expenses aimed at health and social services. Isn't life expectancy in good health more important than life expectancy (WHO 1997)?

Choices to be Made

It is reasonable to believe that tomorrow's elderly will be very different from today's elderly (Marcil-Gratton and Légaré 1987), but the extra years lived compared to their parents raise some questions. Will they be more autonomous? Surely they will on some grounds (emotional, financial, etc.), but as for health, the situation is not as clear. More autonomy in old age implies less years lived with a disability.

To reach such an objective, biomedical research must concentrate its efforts on the prevention of ailments that create the highest rate of chronic disability. This approach towards sicknesses of the elderly puts into question the orientation of biomedical research as it stands. Given the limited resources, are we prepared to re-allocate research funds, both for fundamental as well as applied research, towards illnesses that are not life-threatening? There is surely room here also for numerous technological innovations.

We must also question the use of non-palliative costly health care methods that only succeed in prolonging the suffering of the elderly, for both economic and ethical reasons. We should not ignore the elderly; rather, we should concentrate on more humane care that better corresponds to the needs of the patients, allowing them if not to die in health, then at least to die in dignity (Somers 1988). Clearly, this is only valuing the definition of equity: "To each according to his needs." This should not be interpreted as an attempt jo justify additional budgetary cutbacks to the health care system and biomedical research, but rather to suggest an overhaul of the resources put at their disposal.

Do the budgets allocated to the health care needs of the elderly as well as the trends in geriatric research reflect the pre-occupations of our population? With mentalities rapidly changing, we believe that people will want to control the end of their lives to the same extent that they control their reproduction (Légaré and Marcil-Gratton 1990; Griffiths 1998). Admittedly, as physicians always maintain, the public would like to see research into health issues intensified. However, it would appear that those who are better informed of what is at stake for the future would rather subscribe to the Fries scenario than to the one proposed by Manton. Dying healthy rather than living longer could be a public health goal, as is, for example, the fight against smoking. Our societies must rapidly take a stand on this paradox[4].

References

Barer ML, Evans RG, Hertzman C (1995) Avalanche or glacier? Health care and the demographic rhetoric. Can J Aging 14:193-224

Bodnar AG, Ouellette M, Frolkis M, Holt SE, Chiu CP, Morin GB, Harley CB, Shay JW, Lichtsteiner S, Wright WE (1998) Extension of life-span by introduction of telomerase into normal human cells. Science 279:349-352

Bourbeau R, Légaré J, Emond V (1997) New birth cohort life tables for Canada and Quebec, 1801-1941. Statistics Canada, Demography Division, Demographic Document no. 3, Ottawa (This document can be consulted on Statistics Canada Internet Site: HTTP://www.statcan.ca)

Callahan D (1987) Setting limits: medical goals in an ageing society. Simon and Schuster, New York

Callahan D (1990) What kind of life: the limits of medical progress. Simon and Schuster, New York

Cambois E, Robine JM, Romieu I (1997) Prévalence des incapacités chez les personnes âgées. In Dupaquier J (ed) L'espérance de vie sans incapacités: faits et tendances, premières tentatives d'explication. PUF, Paris pp 121-132

Caselli G, Vallin J (1990) Mortality and population ageing. Eur J Pop Stud 6:1-25

Cribier F (1997) Changement social et allongement de la durée de vie. In: Dupaquier J (ed) L'espérance de vie sans incapacités: faits et tendances, premières tentatives d'explication. PUF, Paris pp 137-149

Crimmins EM, Saito Y, Ingegneri D (1997) Trends in disability-free life expectancy in the United States, 1970-1990. Pop Devel Rev 23:555-572

Druet PP (1990) Les défis éthiques de la société vieillie. In: Loriaux M, Remy D, Vilquin E (eds) Populations âgées et révolution grise. Les hommes et les sociétés face à leurs vieillissements. Editions CIACO, Louvain-La-Neuve, pp 1105-1112

Duchene J, Wunsch G (1988) From the demographer's cauldron: single decrement life tables and the span of life. Genus XLIV:1-17

Egidi V, Frova L (1997) Morbidity, mortality and health-related quality of life in developed countries: concepts, methods and indicators. In: International population conference Beijing 1997. Volume 1, IUSSP, Liège, pp 297-316

Felder S, Meier M (1996) Demand for health care services in the last two years of life. University of Zurich, Zurich

Fries JF (1980) Aging, natural death and the compression of morbidity. New Engl J Med 303:130-135

---

[4] A paradox, according to its Greek etymology, paradoxos, is an idea that goes against opinion, against common sense, against the expected; in brief, an idea in principle which shakes commonly accepted opinion.

Fries JF (1984) The compression of morbidity: miscellaneous comments about a theme. The Gerontologist 24:354–359

Fuch VR (1984) Though much is taken: reflections on aging, health and medical care. Milbank Quart 62:143–166

Gallagher J (1987) Economic limits and bioethics. In: Aging with limited resources. Proceedings of a colloquium on health care, May 1986. Canada Minister of Supply and Services, Ottawa pp 141–144

Griffiths J (1998) Euthanasia and law in the Netherlands. Amsterdam University Press and University of Michigan Press, Amsterdam

Kunitz SJ (1987) Ideologies and explanations of mortality decline. Pop Devel Rev 13:379–408

Kunitz SJ (1991) The personal physician and the historic decline of mortality. In: Schofield R, Reher D, Bideau A (eds) The decline of mortality in Europe. Clarendon Press, Oxford, pp 248–262

Kuntzmann F (1997) Apport de la médecine à l'espérance de vie sans invalidité. In: Dupaquier J (ed) L'espérance de vie sans incapacités: faits et et tendances, premières tentatives d'explication. PUF, Paris pp 179–189

Légaré J, Carrière Y (1991) Mourir en santé plutôt que vivre plus longtemps: un choix de société. In: Durand G, Perrotin C (eds) Contribution à la réflexion bioéthique; dialogue France-Québec. Montréal, Editions Fides. pp 145–164. (Coll. Vie, santé et valeurs)

Légaré J, Marcil-Gratton N (1990) Individual programming of life events: a challenge for demographers in the twenty-first century. Ann NY Acad Sci 610:98–105

Manga P (1987) The allocation of health care resources: ethical and economic choice, conflicts and compromise. Commission d'enquête sur les services de santé et les services sociaux. Synthèse Critique, Québec 33

Manton KG (1982) Changing concepts of morbidity and mortality in the elderly population. Milbank Quart 60:183–244

Manton KG (1991) New biotechnologies and the limits to life expectancy. In: Lutz W (ed) Future demographic trends in Europe and North America. What can we assume today? Academic Press, New York, pp 97–115

Marcil-Gratton N, Légaré J (1987) Being old today and tomorrow: a different proposition. Can Stud Pop 14:237–241

Myers GC (1988) Chronic non-life threatening health aliments. An overlooked dimension. In: Bui DHD (ed) The future of health and health care systems in the industrialized societies. Praeger, New York, pp 67–80

Myers GC, Manton KG (1984) Compression of mortality: myth or reality? The Gerontologist 24:346–353

Rawls J (1971) A theory of justice. Harvard University Press, Boston

Robine JM, Romieu I, Cambois E, van de Water HPA, Boshuizen HC, Jagger C (1995) Global assessment in positive health. INSERM-REVES, Montpellier

Roos NP, Montgomery P, Roos LL (1987) Health care utilization in the years prior to death. Milbank Quart 65:231–254

Schneider EL, Brody JA (1983) Aging, natural death and the compression of morbidity: Another view. New Engl J Med 309:854–856

Schneider EL, Guralnick M (1987) The compression of morbidity: a dream which may come true, some day! Gerontol Persp 1:8–14

Somers AR (1988) Aging in the 21st century: projections, personal preferences, public policies. A consumer view. Healthy Pol 9:49–58

Thatcher AR (1999) The long term pattern of adult mortality and the highest attained age. J Royal Statistical Soc A 162 Part 1 (forthcoming)

Walford RL (1983) Maximum life span. W.W. Norton, New York

WHO (1997) World Health Report 1997. WHO, Geneva

Wilkins R (1987) Is it reasonable to expect a compression of morbidity in the future? Gerontol Persp 1:14–16

Wilkins R, Adams OB (1983) Health expectancy in Canada, late 1970: demographic, regional and social dimensions. Am J Publ Health 73:1073–1080

Wilkins R, Adams OB (1987) Changes in the healthfulness of life of the elderly population: an empirical approach. J Epidemiol Publ Health 35:225–235

Subject index

DATE DUE

SEP 0 9 2009			
APR 2 0 2000			